OXFORD ENGLISH FOR CAREERS

MEDICINE ②

Sam McCarter

Student's Book

D1232907

OXFORD
UNIVERSITY PRESS

Contents

Unit									
7 Dermatology • p.66	Understanding exactly what the patient says	Managing skin conditions	Listening for details / Dealing with teenagers	Applied anatomy and physiology	Skin conditions / Diagnosis and management of skin conditions	Reflection on personal experience	Commenting on the past / Verbs with *to* and *-ing*	Lesions	Main stress in a sentence
Zahra El-Ashry – practice nurse									
8 Surgery • p.74	Putting yourself in the patient's shoes	Post-op pain management / OSCE exams	Patient response / Getting into conversations	Ovarian cysts: What are the symptoms, problems, and possible complications?	Explaining treatments / An ovarian cyst	Describing a complicated operation	Relative pronouns in explanations	Medical terminology for surgery / Technical vocabulary	Secondary stress
9 Cardiology • p.82	Talking to an anxious partner / Competition / Giving advice and coaxing	Cardiac risk factors / Treatment for hypertension and cholesterol	A heart condition / Advice about lifestyle changes	High blood pressure – hypertension	Taking a history / Medication for hypertension	Difficulties in persuasion	The future	Avoidance of technical terms	Speaking at natural speed
10 Respiratory medicine • p.90	Lung conditions	Inhalers	Signs and symptoms / Mistake recognition / Explaining a device	Flow–volume loop	Causes of breathlessness / Explaining tests / Describing a peak flow meter / Explaining an inhaler	Describing data	The definite and indefinite article	Coughs / Nature of the sputum	
11 Tropical diseases • p.98	Positioning and support of a stroke patient	Milestones in public health	Treating returning travellers / Maintaining good health	Sickle-cell anaemia	Developments in public health / Describing a disease / Speaking in group work settings / Patient cultural background	Describing a life cycle	Linking words	Travellers' diarrhoea	
12 Technology • p.106		Technological advances / Trying to persuade the doctor		Stem cell transplant	Controversial developments / Reluctant patients / Stem cell therapy	Stem cell therapy	Negative questions	Change / Evaluating change	

1 Emergency medicine

Check up

1 Work in groups. Describe the type of rapid response shown in the photos.

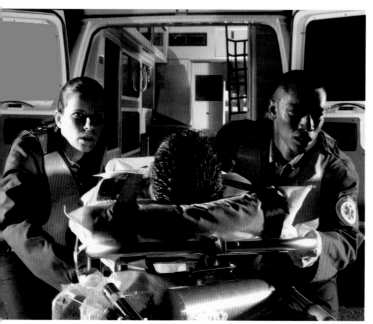

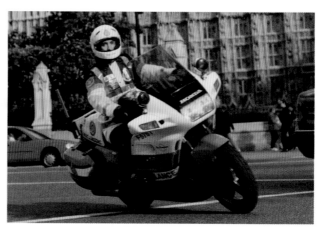

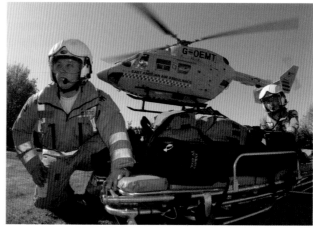

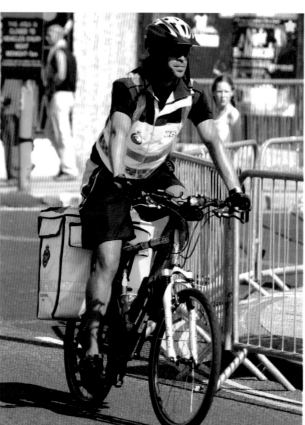

2 Which of these is more appropriate for urban or built-up areas? For rural areas? Give reasons and examples.

3 Which type of response is common in your country?

4 Does working in such areas of medicine appeal to you?

Listening 1

Listening for detail

1 🎧 Listen to a conversation between a doctor and a patient. Write down as many details as you can about what you hear. Compare your answers with a partner.

2 Complete a copy of the form on page 115.

3 🎧 Listen to the conversation again and then compare notes again.

4 Check your details with the rest of the class.

Vocabulary

Adverbs: describing how things happened

1 Adverbs can help to describe how things happened and help to make a diagnosis. Look at these statements from *Listening* 1 and underline the adverbs.

... when suddenly Barbara, my wife, just fainted. We tried to get her upright and she started twitching quite violently.

2 Underline the most appropriate adverb in these sentences.

1 The fainting? It just happened *abruptly / gradually / slowly*. The next thing I knew she was lying completely flat on the pavement.
2 The patient suddenly became pale and started to sweat, but not *profusely / rapidly / enormously*.
3 After the attack, Mr Jones came to *rapidly / slowly / leisurely*, which questions whether it was a seizure.
4 *Embarrassingly / Gradually / Clearly*, I soiled myself and wet myself. It wasn't very pleasant.
5 She was lying flat, but bystanders were trying to keep her upright, so she was twitching *slowly / convulsively / suddenly*.
6 As he couldn't see *good / clearly / visually*, he got quite frightened.
7 In a seizure, there is *typically / rarely / seldom* no prodrome, but this is not always the case.
8 After collapsing, he didn't get better *spontaneously / slowly / gradually*. The patient was a bit drowsy for quite a while afterwards.
9 He recovered *completely / partially / poorly* from the accident. Now he's perfectly OK.
10 Fainting and vomiting don't *reliably / partially / clearly* discriminate seizures from faints.

3 Work in pairs. Decide whether the statements in 2 are likely to be said by a patient or a medical professional.

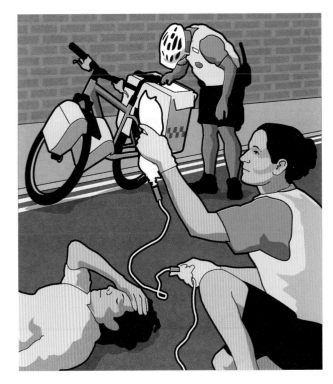

Patient care

1 Decide whether these items are technical or non-technical. Then match them with corresponding words and phrases in *Vocabulary* 2.

a post-ictal
b fit
c to be incontinent of stool
d syncope
e a warning sign
f to be incontinent of water
g supine
h to go into spasm, but not really jerking
i to tell the difference (between)

2 Ideally, when speaking to a patient, you should use non-technical words. Sometimes, you can make the mistake of using technical words. Work in pairs and practise giving lay terms or your own explanations for the technical words above.

EXAMPLE
PATIENT: *I'm sorry, but what's a prodrome? What does supine mean?*
DOCTOR: *It's a ... It means ... It's where ...*

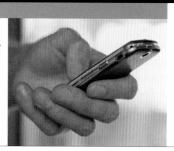

come over (v) suddenly feel
999 (n) the number dialled for emergency calls in the UK

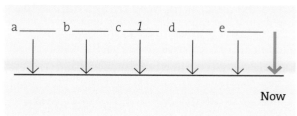

Speaking

Work in pairs. Study the information in the form you completed for *Listening 1*. Take turns role-playing a doctor asking questions to elicit the information from the patient who fainted in the street.

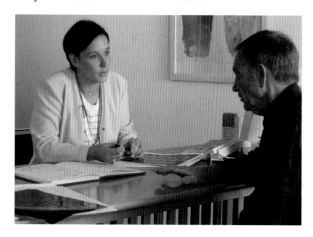

● Language spot

Rapid tense change

1 Understanding the sequence of events and hence the tenses is important for correct diagnosis. What are the tenses of the highlighted phrases?

¹We were shopping in Cambridge Street in town, when suddenly Barbara, my wife, ²just fainted. ³We tried to get her upright and ⁴she started twitching quite violently. ⁵It was quite scary. ⁶She came round very rapidly. But ⁷we dialled 999 and a paramedic appeared almost instantly and then the ambulance almost immediately afterwards. ⁸She had been complaining of feeling a bit unwell, and ⁹had almost fainted and ¹⁰she felt a bit woozy. ¹¹She was a bit dizzy and ¹²she was yawning repeatedly and then all of a sudden, ¹³there she was, lying on the ground. When I come to think of it, ¹⁴she passed out once before about a month ago. ¹⁵She hasn't been feeling well on and off over the summer. ¹⁶We thought it was the heat.

a Present Perfect (Pres Perf)
b Past Continuous (PC)
c Past Perfect (Past Perf)
d Past Perfect Continuous (Past Perf Cont)
e Present Perfect Continuous (Pres Perf Cont)
f Simple Past (SP)

2 Place sentences 1, 2, 8, 9, and 15 on the timeline.

```
a _____ b _____ c _1_ d _____ e _____
  ↓        ↓        ↓        ↓        ↓        ↓
                                          Now
```

3 Complete the sentences using the verbs in brackets in the correct past tense.

1 We _____ (walk) along the street when she _____ (pass) out suddenly.

2 She _____ (have never) the pain before till now, but she _____ (experience) some bleeding the first time.

3 After he _____ (admit), he _____ (become) suddenly worse, but he's started responding to treatment.

4 He _____ (never suffer) a fit before, but he _____ (feel) unwell since this morning.

5 He _____ (yawn) repeatedly, which he _____ (not do) before, and then he just _____ (faint).

6 After he _____ (fall), he _____ (start) twitching violently when we _____ (try) to get him up.

7 When she _____ (lie) on the ground, she _____ (not shake) at all. Then she just stood up.

8 What actually _____ (happen) when she _____ (fall)?

9 He _____ (bite) his tongue and he _____ (mess) himself and he _____ (feel) a bit groggy since.

button battery (n) a small round flat battery

4 Use each of the tenses in brackets once only as you expand these notes into sentences.

1 We eat in a restaurant. I suddenly feel woozy. I faint. This never happen before. (*SP, SP, PC, Pres Perf*)

2 Ahmed never be ill before but feel unwell yesterday. He abruptly cried and then pass out. (*Past Perf, SP, SP*)

3 We travel by train to the city. He not eat since the morning. He vomit and we come straight here. (*SP, Past Perf, SP, PC*)

4 Mary have fainting fits for the past few days. She do a lot of running around when it happen second time. She never have them before. And none of us have them, either. (*PC, Pres Perf Cont, Pres Perf, SP, Pres Perf*)

5 She get out bed when she come over all giddy, but she have it before, so we think nothing of it. (*SP, SP, Past Perf, PC*)

5 Work in pairs and describe your day so far, pointing out

- what you have done so far today
- things you haven't done yet
- things you were doing while doing something else
- and things you had done before you did something.

6 Role-play these situations.

1 Student A, go to page 114. Student B, take a history from Student A. Write notes as you listen and decide what the patient's complaint is.

2 Student B, go to page 116. Student A, take a history from Student B.

» Go to **Grammar reference** p 118

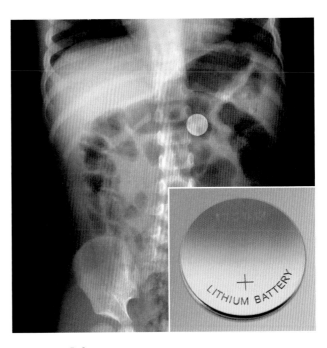

Speaking

1 Work in groups. Decide what would be the main signs and symptoms you would expect in a case

1 where an otherwise fit 30-year-old man presents with pneumonia at A&E **or**

2 where a mother presents at A&E with a child who has swallowed a **button battery**.

2 You are going to role-play the history. Decide which *two* of these items you want to focus on in the assessment of the role-play. Give reasons for your choice.

- the sequence of the tenses
- the grammatical accuracy of the tenses
- the accuracy of the description elicited by the doctor
- the use of non-technical language
- fluency

3 Work with a partner from another group. Each choose one of the two scenarios in **1**. Agree on the two items you want to be assessed on. Take a history from your patient. The patient should make a few notes about the doctor's performance. When you have finished, give feedback to your partner about your own performance and then invite comments from your partner. Remember to begin with positive comments and use constructive criticism.

traffic-busting (adj) able to get through road congestion

free up (v) release

It's my job

1 What do you think the work of a cycle paramedic involves? What do you think are the advantages of a cycle paramedic compared to a conventional ambulance?

2 Work in pairs. Skim the text and the questions in **3** quickly and decide what the text is about.

3 Answer the questions.
1 Do cycle paramedics in London's West End arrive at the scene as rapidly as or more rapidly than conventional ambulances?
2 Is the paramedic's bike equipped with only a basic First Aid Kit or more sophisticated equipment?
3 In serious cases, are the conventional ambulance and the cycle paramedics sent simultaneously or are the latter sent first?

4 Is the bike the most efficient rapid response means or is this not mentioned?
5 Does the cycle paramedic response time in the West End exceed or equal the government benchmark?

4 Work in groups. Is the emergency system similar in your own country? Give examples. How do you think the system described below could operate in urban / rural areas in your country?

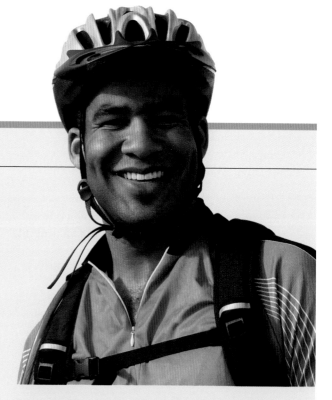

John Rhys

My name is John Rhys, and I'm one of a team of four cycle paramedics of the London Ambulance Service's traffic-busting bicycle ambulance service. We attend 999 emergency calls in the City of London – the financial centre called the Square Mile. The bike itself is the same as those used by the successful cycle units operating in London's West End, which regularly reach patients faster than conventional ambulances.

The team's bikes are fitted with blue lights and sirens, carry a range of equipment, including a heart-starting defibrillator, oxygen, pain-relieving gas, and even a maternity pack for delivering babies.

Where the patient is believed to be in a life-threatening condition, we are sent at the same time as a regular ambulance crew so that we can start treatment before they arrive. Where the patient is understood to be suffering from a more minor injury or illness, we are initially sent on our own and then are able to request further assistance – freeing up ambulances to attend other, more potentially life-threatening, 999 calls elsewhere in the City.

More than 300,000 people work in the City of London and their numbers are swelled by the several million tourists who visit the area each year. Using the bike gives us an opportunity to save potentially vital seconds in starting treatment, especially in the narrow streets which we can negotiate more quickly and easily than ambulances. For example, my colleagues in the West End Cycle Response Unit regularly reach 100 per cent of the most serious, 'Category A', 999 calls within eight minutes. This response is much quicker than the government standard for this category of call of 75 per cent.

Guidelines published by the American Heart Association state that for every minute of delay in getting to a patient in cardiac arrest, the chances of successful resuscitation decrease by 10 per cent.

• Language spot

Comparative and superlative adjectives and adverbs

1 Look at *It's my job.* Can you find examples of comparative and superlative adjectives and adverbs?

EXAMPLE

... reach patients <u>faster</u> than conventional ambulances

2 Complete the sentences with a word from the list. Add any necessary words to indicate comparative or superlative and make any necessary changes to the adjective or adverb.

drowsy	frequent	lively	long	
bad	serious	shallow	violent	wet

1 This time Jessica took _____ to improve than before.

2 She didn't twitch as _____ as the last time.

3 It's _____ I have ever had. It was agony.

4 Is this attack _____ than the last time, or not as bad?

5 He's _____ than he was about ten minutes ago. He's coming to gradually.

6 Natalia appears a bit _____ than the last time we saw her. She's running around.

7 How have you been coping with the weather? It's much _____ than last year.

8 Her breathing is _____ than before.

9 People seem to be coming in with this _____ than last year.

3 Expand the part of the sentences in italics adding a comparative or superlative in each case. In some sentences, both *more* and *less* may be used.

1 He is much *big the last time* you brought him to see us.

2 This is by far *good hospital* I have ever been in.

3 How does this compare to *severe pain* you've had?

4 It's *easy to walk now* it was before the operation.

5 He was sweating *profusely* before.

6 His heart is beating *irregularly* before. It's almost back to normal.

7 I'm pleased. John is *stressed* he was last year.

8 He needs *exercise* to get the full movement back.

4 Work in pairs. Compare your life now as a student / worker with the past. Use these adjectives / adverbs: *hard / easy; stimulating / dull; relaxing / stressful; complicated / simple.* Give reasons and examples.

>> Go to **Grammar reference** p 118

Listening 2

Description of an emergency incident

1 Look at the picture and describe the equipment. What do you think is the benefit of such equipment on cycle ambulances?

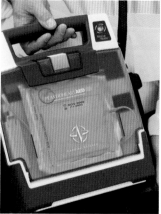

2 🎧 Listen to a case study about an incident at Heathrow Airport. Write down as much detail as you can. Compare notes with a partner.

3 🎧 Listen again and write down the verb only in each missing step.

1 Gary Edwards had been relaxing.

2 He developed a severe pain in his chest and arms.

3 _____

4 His respiration ceased.

5 _____

6 _____

7 A cycle paramedic arrived faster than the ambulance.

8 He continued resuscitation.

9 _____

10 Paramedics, dispatched in an ambulance, turned up a few minutes later.

11 _____

4 Work in pairs and complete the rest of the missing details.

5 In groups, discuss whether this type of rapid response would work in your country. Give reasons and examples.

instigate (v) start

Reading

1 Answer these questions.

1 Do you try to keep up to date with current developments in medicine? How?
2 Is it important to continue studying throughout your medical career? Why?
3 Look at the title. What do you think Continuing Professional Development involves?

2 Find words in the text which have the same meaning as these words.

1 experienced, gone through
2 put together, drafted, compiled, composed
3 altered, changed, modified
4 set up, introduced, started
5 lying behind, underpinning
6 pertinent, applicable
7 requirements, what you require

3 Correct these statements about the text by changing or removing words.

1 All doctors keep a written log of their CPD.
2 The College of Emergency Medicine instigated the process of appraisal.
3 The GMC document *Good Medical Practice* (2001) contributed considerably to the revision of the College guidelines on CPD.
4 CPD is a process that replaces formal education and training.
5 The responsibility for keeping up to date lies with the College of Medicine.

Guidelines on Continuing Professional Development

The vast majority of Emergency Medicine (EM) doctors practise continuing professional development (CPD); however, not all doctors keep a record. CPD has undergone a dramatic evolution and was initially formalized by an agreement in 1993 by the Conference of Medical Royal Colleges and Faculties. The first guidance for continuing medical education (CME) for the College of Emergency Medicine was drawn up in November 1995. Since then there have been many changes due to the introduction of appraisal and recommendations by the GMC (General Medical Council), and the guidelines were amended in January 1999 and January 2000. The most recent edition of the guidelines was written in September 2003.

Since appraisal has been instituted and revalidation is inevitable despite the delay in the implementation, the documentation of proof of CPD has become more relevant.

This revision of the College guidelines on CPD is based on:

- *A framework for Continuing Professional Development* – The Academy of Medical Royal Colleges (February 2002)
- *Guidelines on CPD Faculty of Accident and Emergency Medicine* – Henry Guly, past Director of CPD (2003)
- *The GMC guidelines on CPD* (April 2004)
- The GMC document *Good Medical Practice* (2001)

Principles underlying Continuing Professional Development

Continuing Professional Development (CPD) is a continuing learning process that complements formal undergraduate and postgraduate education and training. CPD requires you to maintain and improve your standards across all areas of your practice. CPD should also encourage and support specific changes in your practice and career development.

CPD is an obligatory requirement for all practising Emergency Medicine physicians and it is up to each doctor [you] to keep up to date.

The GMC set out in paragraph 10 of *Good Medical Practice* (September 2001)

'You must keep your knowledge and skills up to date throughout your working life. In particular, you should take part regularly in educational activities which maintain and further develop your competence and performance.'

However, CPD must be relevant to you and meet your needs to allow maintenance of a high quality of patient care. Continuing professional development should be reflective, lifelong learning allowing you to develop within the specialty of emergency medicine, and should also support you in developing outside or subspecialty interests.

[CPD Guidance GMC April 2004]

Project

1 Work in groups. Are jobs in A&E departments / Emergency departments popular in your country? Why / Why not?

2 What methods are common in your country for obtaining jobs, e.g. recruitment by job advert, curriculum vitae (CV) followed by an interview?

3 What do you understand by a job specification / job spec?

Writing

A job application

1 Look at this extract from a job application form for a post in the emergency department of a large city hospital.

Job application

State why you think you should be considered for this post giving

- suitability for the post
- relevant experience
- training
- qualities

---

2 Write a description of your suitability for the post or a post in your speciality. Remember the information must be individual to you and contain genuine details.

Speaking

In an interview, remember that what you say needs to match accurately what you have written in your job application. Work in pairs. Give your description from your job application in *Writing 2* to a partner. Take turns asking each other about the details you wrote. Check the description for accuracy.

Make sure that what you are saying does not sound as if you have learnt it by heart. Avoid repeating exactly what you have written.

USEFUL EXPRESSIONS
When I was in ...
After I finished ...
What makes me suitable for the post is ...
The relevant experience I have is ...
I've followed various training courses like ...
As regards my qualities, ...

Checklist

Assess your progress in this unit.
Tick (✓) the statements which are true.

- I can change tenses rapidly
- I can understand adverbs of manner
- I can do third party interviewing
- I can understand comparison
- I can understand continuing professional development

Key words

Adverbs
abruptly
embarrassingly
spontaneously

Nouns
appraisal
bystander
Continuing Professional Development
job specification
paramedic
rapid response
seizure
warning sign

Adjectives
giddy
groggy
woozy

Verbs
dispatch
faint
soil
twitch
wet

Useful reference

Oxford Handbook of Emergency Medicine
3rd edition, Wyatt et al,
ISBN 978-0-19-920607-0

2 Accidents

Check up

1 Describe the pictures.

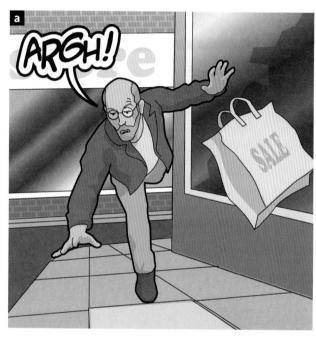

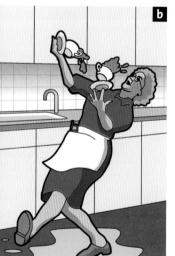

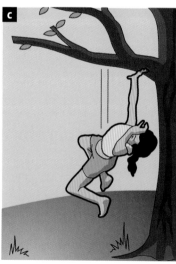

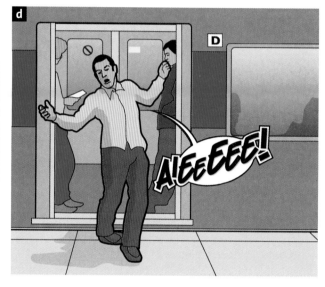

2 What type(s) of injuries do you think can occur in each case?

3 Are these accidents preventable? Why / Why not?

Vocabulary

Fractures

1 Match the descriptions 1–8 with the types of fracture a–h.

1 simple
2 avulsion
3 spiral
4 comminuted
5 crush
6 stress
7 impacted
8 hairline

a which occurs when certain bones are likely to break from repeated minor injuries

b where the ends of a bone are driven into each other

c a complex fracture which results in more than two bone fragments

d where the volume of bone is reduced because it has been compressed

e where there is a single fracture of the bone with only two main fragments

f where a bit of bone is pulled off with a ligament or muscle

g which is not very clear and there is no clear displacement

h which is seen in long bones as a result of twisting injuries

2 Work in pairs. Describe a fracture to your partner, who then gives the name.

In this unit
● knowledge about fractures
● describing fractures and accidents
● Present Simple, Present Continuous, Present Perfect
● giving instructions with the imperative and *need*

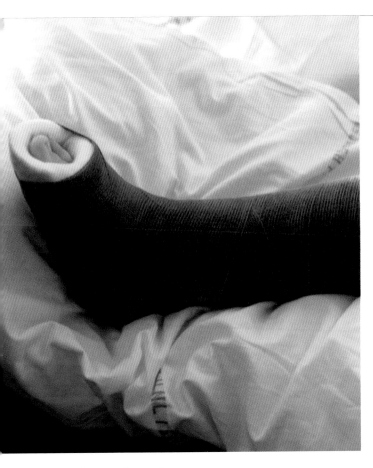

Listening 1

Understanding verb tenses

1 🎧 Listen and match each conversation with a picture in *Check up*.

1 ＿＿＿

2 ＿＿＿

3 ＿＿＿

2 🎧 Listen again and write down the tenses (a–c) of the verbs as they occur in each conversation.

a Present Simple
b Present Continuous
c Present Perfect

1		2		3	
hurt	＿＿	hurt	＿＿	cry	＿＿
give	＿＿	break	＿＿	fracture	＿＿
happen	＿＿	look	＿＿		

● Language spot

Talking about the present

1 🎧 You are going to hear three statements by either a doctor or a patient. Listen and decide who is speaking and what they are talking about.

2 🎧 Listen again and write down the order in which the tenses are used.

1 Present Continuous ＿＿＿ Present Simple ＿＿＿
Present Perfect ＿＿＿

2 Present Continuous ＿＿＿ Present Simple ＿＿＿
Present Perfect ＿＿＿

3 Present Continuous ＿＿＿ Present Simple ＿＿＿
Present Perfect ＿＿＿

3 In your own words explain why each tense is being used in the three statements.

4 Read the statements made by patients and doctors. One tense in each item is wrong. Which one is it?

1 I just slam the door on my finger and it's bleeding a lot. It's really painful.

2 The X-ray is coming back and it shows you have a hairline fracture here and here. Is it hurting you at the moment?

3 Yes, the doctor's given me a telephone number and written instructions in case anything is happening with the plaster cast. But honestly, I'm fine. I'm not getting pins and needles or anything like that.

4 Yes, I've seen the doctor and he's given me some painkillers. I've just waited for the nurse to come back. When she comes back, I can go home.

5 It mends rather nicely, considering you have had a rather nasty fall. But avulsion fractures heal quite well.

6 Are you wearing your neck brace all the time? Yes? And do you begin to regain movement?

7 I immobilize his arm with a backslab POP and the X-rays have been done. They demonstrate the whole lengths of the radius and the ulna. I think he's feeling comfortable.

>> Go to **Grammar reference** p 119

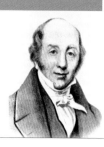

Abraham Colles, 1773–1843,
Professor of Surgery, Dublin

Vocabulary

Causes of injury

1 Complete the sentences using the verbs below.

banged	dislocated	fell	landed
pulled	slipped	smash	squashed
stubbed	stumbled	tripped	twisted
twisted	went over		

1 I _____ on a loose paving stone as I was walking down the street and _____ flat on my face.

2 I _____ and lost my footing and _____ my ankle.

3 I _____ my toe on a chair. I may have fractured it, but I hope I haven't.

4 I _____ my knee on the metal table. I am surprised I didn't _____ my kneecap to pieces.

5 I _____ my ankle when I went over and now I can barely walk. I don't think it's broken or anything. It's more likely to be a sprain.

6 I _____ on the wet floor and went over and _____ on my bottom.

7 The motorbike _____ on my ankle and crushed my leg.

8 I think I've _____ my shoulder and I can barely move it.

9 I _____ my finger in the door and it's throbbing like mad.

10 I _____ this nick out of the side of my fingernail and now it's infected.

2 Work in pairs. Have you ever treated someone who has injured themselves as in **1** above? Describe the case.

Speaking

1 Look at the X-rays. Identify the type of fracture for patients a and b.

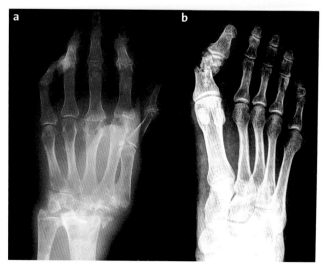

2 Work in pairs. Choose an X-ray and create a history for the patient. Include these details: name, sex, age, the presenting complaint (what the problem is, how / where / when it happened, etc.), need of analgesia, and any other details you wish to add.

3 Work with a partner from another pair with a different scenario and take the history up to the point of sending the patient for an X-ray.

4 Explain the X-ray to the patient.

It's my job

1 Work in pairs. What do you think the job of a radiologist involves? How has the radiologist's work changed in the last half century?

2 Read the text and answer the questions.

1 Where did Matthew Jenkins originally find that radiology appealed to him?

2 How does he describe the Royal College's booklet?

3 What is the main purpose of radiology?

4 What does the radiologist see as his role?

5 Why is it important to include the details mentioned on the request form?

6 Why is the radiologist's day busy?

I am glad to say that in this country there is no need to carry out tests as a form of insurance. It is not in this country desirable, or indeed necessary, that overprotective and over examination work should be done merely and purely as I say to protect oneself against possible litigation.
– *Judge Fallon, quoted by Oscar Craig, Chairman Cases Committee, Medical Protection Society.*
– *Oxford Handbook of Emergency Medicine*

Matthew Jenkins

My name is Matthew Jenkins and I am a radiologist at a hospital in Manchester. I decided to take up radiology as a specialty after working in various other departments first. It was in the A&E department that my interest was first aroused. I was at a loss initially as a young doctor out of medical training as to how to make a request to the radiology department even for something as basic as an X-ray. But I soon found my feet. A very useful guide for doctors is the Royal College of Radiologists' booklet, *Making the Best Use of a Department of Clinical Radiology*, (5th edition, London 2003). This is a must-have for doctors dealing with radiology departments and is highly recommended.

The primary aim of radiology is to provide information in order to alter the management of the patient and the outcome of the disease. So my function as a radiologist is to help confirm a diagnosis, exclude something important, define the extent, and monitor the progress of a disease. Most of the requests for X-rays that we receive in the department now come though electronically rather than face-to-face with a clinician. It is therefore important that all relevant clinical information including the mechanism of the injury with the side involved, blood tests, recent radiological findings, and suspected clinical diagnosis is given on the request form. Without the benefit of being able to examine the patient, all of this detail is crucial.

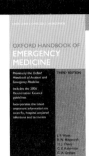

Forms should also state how the investigation will help resolve the clinical problem facing the doctor and state any investigations on the request form if the doctor thinks they will take place.

Each day my schedule is full as I try to balance the needs and priorities of different departments.

3 Work in groups. Do you think the radiologist's job will become less or more complex in the future? Give reasons and examples.

4 Describe a situation where a radiologist helped you in your work.

Writing

Describing a fracture

1 Complete the list of the information which is needed to describe a fracture.

1 the age of the patient and how the fracture occurred
2 if it is simple or compound
3 name the bone
4 describe the position of the fracture (proximal, supracondylar)
5 _____
6 _____
7 _____
8 _____
9 _____

2 Match the different elements to this description.

29-year-old male motorcyclist with a Type I compound fractured left humerus. It is minimally displaced and involves the humeral shaft with no neurovascular compromise …

3 Write descriptions for the X-rays in *Speaking* on page 14. In each case the patient is a 40-year-old female police officer.

Speaking

1 Work in groups. Which of these X-rays shows an avulsion fracture? What do the other X-rays show?

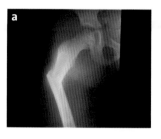

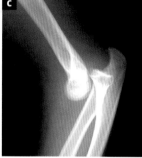

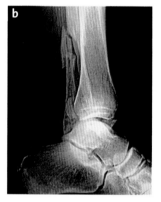

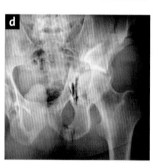

Answers

a Incomplete fracture of the femur in a child
b Avulsion fracture of the ankle
c Pulled elbow
d Hip fracture in an adult

2 Check your answers. Prepare a short presentation of no more than five minutes explaining one or more of the following:

- the X-ray
- the likely causes
- the symptoms
- the treatment.

3 Choose one or more students from your group to present the X-ray to the rest of the class. Make the presentation and invite comments at the end of the presentation.

4 Give constructive feedback for each presentation, choosing two of these criteria: *organization, relevance, fluency, clinical accuracy, grammatical accuracy.*

Reading

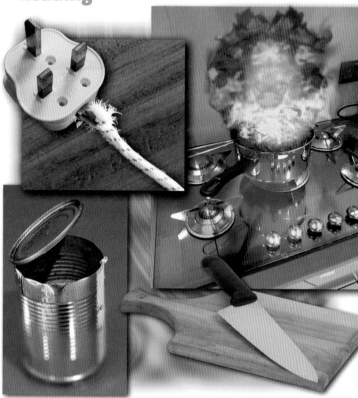

1 Before you read the text, answer the questions.

1 Where do you think the majority of accidents occur: the home, work, or in the street?
2 Which groups of society are more prone to accidents?
3 Are accidents at work generally preventable?

2 Skim the text and match the headings with the appropriate paragraph A–D.

1 Accidents in the home
2 Accidents in the workplace
3 Accidents and children
4 Accidents and the elderly

3 Find words and phrases in the text which have the same meaning as these. Items 1–7 are not in the order they occur in the text.

1 stated
2 deaths
3 among the poor
4 encouraging
5 as a matter of course
6 weakness
7 attending

pressure sore (n) decubitus ulcer
multifactorial (adj) involving many
features or elements
chip pan fires (n) fires created from
cooking chipped potatoes in hot fat

4 Answer the questions about the text.
  1 Among children, which group had the greatest mortality rate?
  2 Among which group are accidents more frequent?
  3 What kind of help should be offered to the elderly who are susceptible to falls?
  4 What are the main sources of accidental fires in homes?
  5 What are doctors responsible for averting?

Accidents

A In 2004, there were 230 child fatalities due to accidents in England and Wales, the highest numbers being in five- to fourteen-year-olds. The commonest cause of accidental injury in children presenting to UK hospitals is falls. Others include suffocating and choking, burns and scalds, and poisoning. A recent report by the Audit Commission and the Healthcare Commission states that each year there are two million attendances to accident and emergency departments by children as a result of accidents that might have been prevented. Accidents are more common in the lower socio-economic groups.

B Frailty and health problems make the elderly, particularly those over the age of 75, at increased risk of accidents, usually occurring in the home. Falls are the most common cause. Inability to get up after falling puts the person at risk of hypothermia and pressure sores. Hip fractures after falls are a major cause of morbidity and mortality.

NICE guidelines were issued in 2004 on the assessment and prevention of falls in older people. They state that older people should be asked routinely if they have fallen in the past year. Those who have fallen, or those considered at risk of falling, should have a multifactorial falls risk assessment and should be considered for interventions including those to improve their strength and balance and remove any home hazards.

C In England and Wales in 2004, there were 3,892 accidental deaths in and around the home. Those most at risk of serious or fatal injury in the home are young children and the elderly. Falls are the most common type of accident.

In 2004, fire brigades attended 442,700 fires in the UK. There were 508 fire-related deaths and 14,600 non-fatal casualties. A large proportion of fires in homes were accidental, the main causes being misuse of equipment / appliances and chip pan fires.

D During 2005 / 2006 there were 148,713 occupational injuries reported, of which 212 were fatal. All places of work are potentially dangerous whether an oil rig, a coal mine, a factory, an office, or a kitchen. The Health and Safety Executive has stipulated rules about safety in the workplace. It also has the necessary powers to inspect and enforce them. Safety equipment must be worn. Risks must be appreciated. Every workplace should have a safety officer who is responsible for identifying danger and advocating action. As doctors, we have a duty to be aware of measures to prevent infection and needle-stick injury.

safety net (n) a reminder to the patient that they can come back if there are any changes or if anything happens

Listening 2

Accident prevention measures

1 🎧 Listen to the extract from a talk on accident prevention measures and tick (✓) the items which are mentioned.

1 _____ Advice about preventing accidents is more the responsibility of the government.

2 _____ When we use the word *accident*, this somehow signifies that something cannot be avoided.

3 _____ Simple safety measures and thinking about the future can reduce accidents.

4 _____ Patients can be alerted to any risky situations.

5 _____ People need to be more aware of accidents caused by leisure than by home improvements.

6 _____ Halls and stairways need to have good lighting.

7 _____ Loose rugs and flooring are dangerous for old people.

2 What other precautions need to be taken at home? Think of the kitchen and heating.

● Language spot

Saying what's necessary politely but firmly

● In certain situations when you are giving patients information, there is not really any negotiation – on discharging a patient or where there is no alternative, for example. In any situation, you need to provide a 'safety net' in case something happens.

You need ... Don't hesitate ...	... to come back and see us if anything unusual happens.
If anything unusual happens, ...	... come back and see us immediately. ... you don't need to ring – just come in.
You need to ... You're going to have to ...	... rest your leg for a while.

Note: avoid using *you have to ...* and *you must ...* (on its own without *if*).

Underline the alternatives in italics which are correct. In some cases, more than one may be correct.

1 If the arm swells in the plaster cast, *come back / you need to come back / you'll come back* and see us.

2 *Don't hesitate to / You are going to / you needn't* contact us if it gets worse in any way.

3 If your fingers become discoloured, *raise / you need to raise / you're going to raise* your hand and try to keep it up.

4 If the plaster cast becomes tight, *you need to come back / come back / try to come back* immediately.

5 If your hand becomes paralysed, *don't wait, just come in / you need to come in / you needn't come in.*

6 If you get any pain in your arm, *don't leave it / you needn't to leave it / you don't need to leave it* – come straight in.

7 If you get any circulation problems like pins and needles, *you need to get / get yourself / don't hesitate to get yourself* back here immediately.

8 If the cast becomes damaged or loose, *replace / we're going to need to replace / we need to replace* it.

▶▶ Go to **Grammar reference** p 120

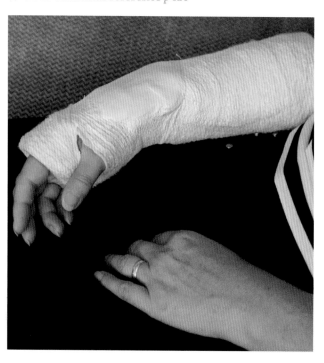

Speaking

1 These six pictures show common minor injuries you might see in an A&E department. Describe the injury shown in each picture.

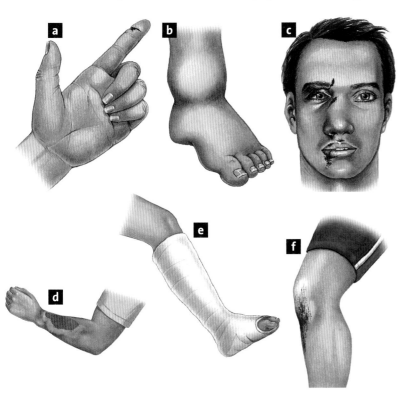

2 Work in groups. Create a history for a nineteen-year-old patient, Gerhard / Gabriele Schneider, who presents with one or more of the above minor injuries. Include

- details about how the injury happened
- when and where it happened
- treatment
- instructions you would give by way of 'safety netting'.

3 Find a partner from another group and indicate the injuries you have according to the history you have created. Take turns taking the history from each other. Use the grid to give feedback about the language used by the doctor.

	Doctor 1	Doctor 2
Uses tenses		
Uses the tenses fluently		
Uses non-technical language		
Uses safety netting		

Checklist

Assess your progress in this unit.
Tick (✓) the statements which are true.

- I can talk about fractures
- I can describe accidents
- I can use the Present Simple, Present Continuous, and Present Perfect
- I can give instructions with the imperative and *need*

Key words

Adjectives
hairline
impacted
prone
simple
spiral

Nouns
avulsion
fracture
POP
safety net

Verbs
bang
dislocate
land
slip (over)
smash
squash
stub
stumble
trip (over / up)
twist

Useful reference

Oxford Handbook of Emergency Medicine
3rd edition, Wyatt et al,
ISBN 978-0-19-920607-0

3 Sports medicine

Check up

1 Describe the pictures.

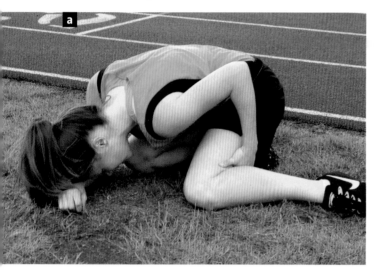

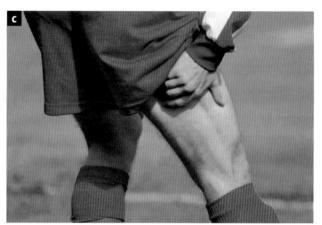

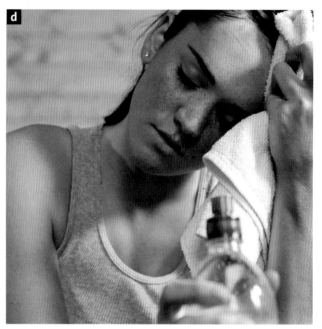

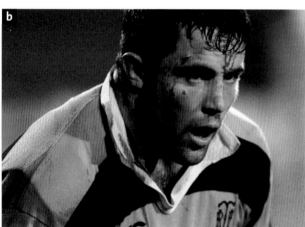

2 Match the lay statements with the pictures in **1**.
   1 I'm covered in cuts and bruises.
   2 I think I've pulled a muscle in my leg.
   3 I've got cramp all down this leg.
   4 I'm dying of thirst.

3 What other injuries are the sportspeople in the pictures prone to? Give examples from your experience.

4 In groups, discuss the questions.
   Are you interested in sports medicine? Why / Why not?
   What are the advantages of following a career in sports medicine? Are there any disadvantages?

Listening 1

Spot the difference

1 🎧 Listen. Write down details of what the patient said. Compare your notes with a partner.

2 🎧 Listen to another version of the same conversation. Which details are different?

3 What is the difference in the questions that the doctor uses in each conversation?

4 Which technique is better for the patient? Which approach do you find easier to use?

Vocabulary

Verbs of movement

1 In conversation **1** in *Listening 1* the doctor was just about to give the patient some instructions. What instructions do you think she might give the patient to check the wrist?

2 Work in groups and match the instructions to the pictures.

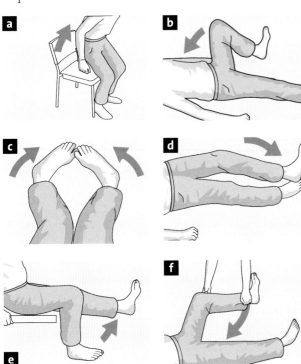

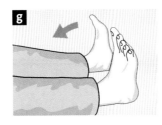

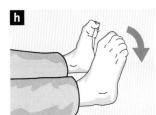

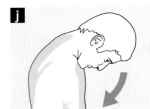

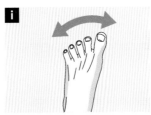

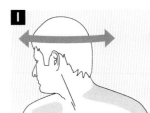

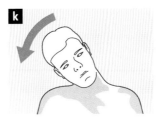

1 Bring your knee towards your chest.
2 Straighten the leg at the knee.
3 Put your chin on your chest.
4 Look over each shoulder.
5 Stand up straight without support.
6 Cross your legs over.
7 Lean your head sideways placing your ear on your shoulder.
8 Point your toes at your head.
9 Fan out your toes as far as possible.
10 Bend the knee as far as you can.
11 Curl your toes and then straighten your toes.
12 Keep your knees together and spread the ankles as far as possible.

3 Work in pairs. You are going to check a patient who has a shoulder injury from the gym. Decide what instructions you would use for the drawings below. Then take turns giving instructions to the patient.

USEFUL EXPRESSIONS
I'd (just) like you to …   *OK.*
Could / can you just … for me?   *Fine.*
I need you to …   *Thank you.*

No class of questions is 'correct'. Sometimes you need to ask one type of question; sometimes another. Get good at shifting from one kind to another and you will soon learn to judge the most important questions for the patient in front of you.
– *Oxford Handbook of Clinical Medicine*

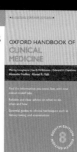

Signs and symptoms
Patient vocabulary

1 Look at the picture. What does it show and what is the colloquial term for these?

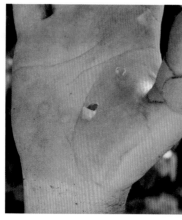

2 Complete the sentences using the words below. You will use one body part more than once. What do the sentences mean?

armpit   back   feet   foot   hand
hands   leg   neck shoulder arm

1 I've got frozen _____. I can't get my arm up very far.

2 I've got wry_____. I can barely move my head.

3 I've got what I think is a boil in my _____. I can't put any deodorant on.

4 I think I've pulled a muscle in my _____. I can only hobble along.

5 I've got these blisters all over the palm of my

_____.

6 I'm not sure but I think I've torn a ligament in my _____. It's swollen and I can't get my shoe on.

7 I've got a lot of calluses on the balls of both

_____.

8 The knuckles on both _____ have all flared up. I can't get my ring off.

9 I've got a pain right here in the small of my

_____.

10 I've got tingling all the way down my left

_____ and _____.

3 Match the medical terms with words and phrases in 2.

(adhesive) capsulitis   bullae   torticollis
furuncle   hyperkeratosis   paraesthesia

● Language spot
Types of questions

1 Use the cues to make questions.

1 Have fall over?
2 Can tell if you trip in the street?
3 you hurt?
4 What think the problem?
5 Who around when pain set in?
6 Could describe what happen me?
7 How long you have chest pain? (Looking at the patient holding his chest)
8 there any other things you like talk about?
9 What else you concern about?
10 the phlegm brown, yellow, or green?

2 Identify the type of question in 1 by using the descriptions. More than one may be possible for each answer.

a a closed question
b an open question
c a leading question
d a patient-centred question
e a family- / work-related question
f a prejudicial question or question suggesting the answer

3 In pairs, work out the questions for these answers. In some cases a prompt has been given. There may be more than one answer in each case.

1 It hurts just here.
2 Well, I don't know where to start really. I suppose it happened just after I had been to ...
3 It's gone completely black.
4 No, not that I am aware of. (trauma: knock / bang)
5 Sitting at my desk at work. (when it's worst)
6 For a week now.
7 No. I can't think of anything.

stand in for (v) replace temporarily, be a locum

4 Use your own words to complete the doctor's questions in the conversation.

DOCTOR Good morning, my name is Dr Nesbitt. I'm standing in for Dr Ratana while he's on holiday. You're Mr Finn?

PATIENT Yes.

DOCTOR OK. 1_____?

PATIENT Well, mmm, I'm not feeling too good.

DOCTOR 2_____?

PATIENT Mmm. I have this pain in my back.

DOCTOR 3_____?

PATIENT A couple of weeks now.

DOCTOR 4_____?

PATIENT Yes. Off and on for a year or so. But never like this.

DOCTOR 5_____?

PATIENT Well, I could barely move at first. And now it's like a dull ache. I just have to be careful getting up and it's not easy at all getting in and out of the car either.

DOCTOR 6_____?

PATIENT Mmm, just here in the small of my back.

DOCTOR 7_____?

PATIENT No. It stays just here.

DOCTOR 8_____?

PATIENT Nothing really, but I can't stay in the one position for long. And walking and lying down hurts too and, well, I suppose ... I usually go to the gym quite a lot.

DOCTOR 9_____?

PATIENT Not since this started.

DOCTOR 10_____?

PATIENT Mmm. Well, I still drive, but getting down into the car is not that easy.

DOCTOR Is it a sports car, then?

PATIENT Yes.

5 Work in groups. Is the conversation patient centred? What type of questions does the doctor ask? Could you improve the conversation?

6 Write out the conversation keeping the same patient information, but changing the doctor's questions where you would like to.

>> Go to **Grammar reference** p 120

Speaking

1 Work in pairs. Role-play Dr Nesbitt (Student A) and take the history from the patient (Student B) in *Language spot* **4** opposite. Remember to be patient centred and ask open questions.

2 Student A, go to page 114. Student B, take a history from Student A. Write notes as you listen and decide what the patient's complaint is.

3 Student B, go to page 116. Student A, take a history from Student B.

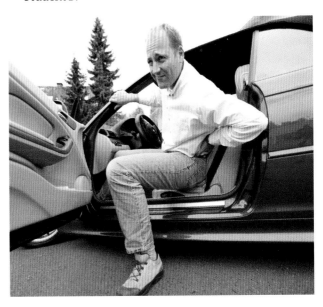

Reading

1 Find adjectives and nouns with similar meaning that are used to describe nouns in the text.

1 related to carrying heavy objects
2 covered many people
3 carried out over a period of time
4 related to contests
5 related to exploring and studying
6 worth noting
7 related to questions about physical activity

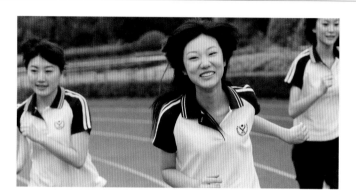

Physical fitness and health

A series of research findings illustrates the positive relationships between physical activity and bone mineral density (BMD) in a variety of sub-populations. In longitudinal studies using various sample sizes, Kemper et al and Puntilla et al illustrate that regular (weight-bearing) physical activity is significantly related to BMD at the lumbar spine and femoral neck. In relation to total body and lumbar spine BMD, van Langendonck et al illustrate that the type of sports participation is a significant factor, with high impact sports (ground forces higher than four times body weight) most effective and remaining beneficial for the skeletal health of males aged 40. Ryan et al report on the effects of six months' whole body resistive training in both young and older men and women. They report that the programme increased muscle mass and improved BMD in the femoral region for all and suggest that if BMD is increased at skeletal maturity, reductions might be achieved in fracture risk in later years. Supporting this conclusion Neville et al demonstrate the importance of sports involving high peak strain for determining peak bone status, especially in young men and possibly for young women (who are less likely to take part in such sports). Greendale et al, in a study of 42- to 52-year-old women, explore four domains of physical activity (sport, home, work, active living). They illustrate that both sport and weight-bearing work in the home were the best, and equal, predictors of greater BMD at lumbar spine and femoral neck sites. The work of Cheng et al raises the one negative note in this literature, finding that high levels of physical activity (running twenty or more miles per week) were associated with osteoarthritis (knee and hip joints) among men less than 50 years of age (although no relationship was suggested among women or older men).

A number of papers address the more general issue of the relationship between sports participation and health behaviours in young people. Miller et al (2000) use data from a large-scale survey of school pupils to illustrate that athletic participation has both positive and negative implications for adolescent health and recommend ways to use sport for health promotion. Pastor et al use survey data on fifteen- to eighteen-year-olds to conclude that the higher the levels of sports participation, the higher the perceived fitness and consequently enhanced perceived health, with lower levels of smoking and alcohol use also enhancing health perceptions. However, the relationships are only weak to moderate. Pyle et al's survey data on high school students illustrate that, for males and females, competitive sports participation was associated with a lower frequency of mental ill-health, eating and dietary problems, and total risks (although there was a higher frequency of sports-related injuries).

2 In the text a number of researchers, e.g. Kemper et al, and the focus of their research are mentioned. Match each description to a researcher.

1 looked only at women
2 explored information on older teenagers only
3 mentioned findings relating to men and running
4 made suggestions to improve health
5 researched both genders over a wide age range

3 Work in groups. Answer the questions.

- How can people be encouraged to participate in sport? Think, for example, of clubs, education, and advertising.
- Is it difficult to dissuade people from over-exercising or exercising when they are injured? What strategies can you use? Can you order or persuade the patient? Give an example of what you would say.

In the sick room, ten cents' worth of human understanding equals ten dollars' worth of medical science.
– *Martin H. Fischer*

Listening 2

Patient attitude

1 Look at the picture. How would you describe the patient's attitude?

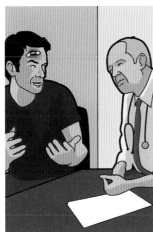

2 Listen to the conversation between Dr Johnston and Mr Alexander Munro. Map the patient's attitude as the conversation progresses by numbering the adjectives.

a ecstatic ☐
b exasperated ☐
c desperate ☐
d annoyed ☐
e uncooperative ☐
f irresponsible ☐
g friendly ☐
h receptive ☐

3 Listen again and do the same for the doctor.

a exasperated ☐   d patient ☐
b cooperative ☐   e persuasive ☐
c calm ☐

4 Listen to the conversation again. Which words are used by the doctor?

1 but you must … ☐
2 we need you to … ☐
3 I'm afraid you do need … ☐
4 You may feel well, but …. ☐
5 I'm sorry but you must … ☐
6 Yes, but other things could happen like … ☐
7 You may get a .. ☐

5 Listen to the conversation again. Which words are used by the patient?

1 You mean I have to stay … ☐
2 but I can't. I have to go to … ☐
3 Oh, thank you. That's kind of you … ☐
4 But I feel OK … ☐
5 I appreciate this … ☐
6 Well, I can take … ☐
7 OK, but I can … ☐

Patient care

1 Look at the following patient's reasons for not following the doctor's instructions after a minor head injury. How would you respond to them?

1 But I'd like to go a friend's birthday party.
2 But can't I just go and ring if I feel bad?
3 But I need to go and pick up my child from school.
4 I'm sorry, but I have no one to be with me for that length of time.
5 If I don't turn up, I'm going to be in trouble with my boss.
6 If I stay in hospital, I'm going to miss an important job interview.
7 And I'll miss the plane. I have to catch a flight to a football match in Germany.
8 And I can't get to sleep without sleeping tablets.

2 Match the replies to the patient's excuses.

a I'm afraid, unless you have someone to be with, we'd need you to …
b You need to avoid them; otherwise you can't be roused.
c And what if you feel dizzy or vomit all of a sudden and …?
d But can't we arrange for your wife or a friend to meet her?
e But if you go to the party, you won't rest and you may be tempted …
f I'm afraid if you go to a game and you don't rest for the next 24 hours, …
g But can you not just phone and rearrange …?
h You need to rest for the next 24 hours rather than exerting yourself working; otherwise, you could be off …

3 Work in pairs. Take turns reading the patient's excuses and replying in your own way.

Pronunciation

Main stress

1 Before you listen, underline the word that you think has the main stress in the part of the sentence in italics.

 1 Can you tell me a little bit more about _how it all happened_?
 2 _But if your child's mood changes in any way_, make sure you contact us immediately.
 3 _But I can't._ I have to go to my best friend's party this evening.
 4 _But I'm afraid you do need to be careful._
 5 I'm not sure _but I think I've torn a ligament in my foot._ It's swollen and I can't get my shoe on.
 6 I've had it since the week before last, _here on the heel of my hand._
 7 _And you need to have someone to go home with you_ and stay with you for the next 24 hours as well.

2 🎧 Listen and mark with a 'O' the syllable in **1** that has the main stress in each clause.

3 Work in pairs. Practise saying the statements to each other and check each other's pronunciation.

4 Make seven questions of your own to take a history from a patient who has fallen off a bicycle and hurt his knee. Use the range of questions in _Language spot_ on page 22.

5 Change partners and take the history. Try not to focus on the pronunciation. Give each other feedback specifically about the pronunciation. You may want to practise taking the history several times.

6 Which statement in **1** has proportionately fewer weak stresses? Why does lay language generally have a larger proportion of weak stresses?

Speaking

1 Work in groups of three. Look at the following example of the head injury warning card for adults. Identify which points the doctor already covered in _Listening 2_ on page 25.

An example of head injury warning instructions

Adults

Ensure a responsible person is available to keep an eye on you for the next 24 hours and show them this card.

Rest for the next 24 hours.

Do take painkillers such as paracetamol to relieve pain and headache.

DO NOT DRINK alcohol for the next 24 hours.

DO take normal medication but DO NOT take sleeping tablets or tranquillizers without consulting your doctor first.

If any of the following symptoms occur, then you should return or be brought back in or the hospital should be telephoned immediately. Tel:********* (24 hours):

- Headache not relieved by painkillers such as paracetamol
- Vomiting
- Disturbance of vision
- Problems with balance
- Fits
- Patient becomes unrousable

2 Take turns role-playing the conversation between Dr Johnston and Alexander Munro from _Listening 2_. The third student uses the speaking checklist on page 117 for the patient and the doctor to give feedback. Use these criteria for assessing the doctor: _able to negotiate, persuasive without being bossy, calm, showing empathy._ Remember to include 'safety netting' at the end.

3 Now work in groups and study this scenario.

Mrs Newman, a 25-year-old mother, brings her seven-year-old child into A&E. The child bumped his head during a Physical Education (PE) class at school. The mother was called and she brought the child in. After a thorough examination you are satisfied that the injury is not serious. Explain to the mother what precautions she needs to take. Note that the mother wants to take the child to a party later in the day.

4 Adapting the advice for adults, make a list of the 'warnings' you give the parent. Remember to include 'safety netting' at the end.

5 Again work in groups of three, role-playing the scenario in **3**. Follow the same procedure as in **2** above. Note that the attitude of the parent is caring and cooperative, but initially she wants to take the child to the party.

Writing

Head injury warning instructions

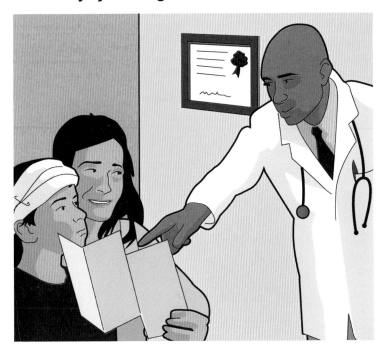

1 Look at the 'head injury warning card' for adults in **1** in *Speaking*. Using this as an example, write 'head injury warning instructions' for a sports centre, to be given to teachers and parents of children who have had a minor head injury while using the sports facilities. Look at these additional points to watch out for:

- child's mood
- behaviour: fits, ...
- cannot rouse
- rest
- tiredness
- safety netting.

2 Write the instructions in groups and share your examples with the class.

3 Role-play the scenario in *Speaking* **3** again. Check for improvements in the light of the instructions you have written.

Key words

Nouns
ball
blister
frozen shoulder
heel
persuasion
small of the back
tingling
warning
wryneck

Adjectives
exasperated
uncooperative

Verbs
bump
curl
fan out
flare up
hobble
negotiate
straighten

Abbreviation
et al

Useful reference

Oxford Handbook of Sport and Exercise Medicine, Domhall MacAuley (ed), ISBN 978-0-19-856839-1

4 Obstetrics

Check up

1 Work in pairs. What do you think is happening in each picture?

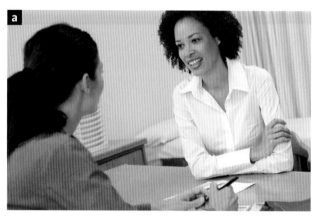

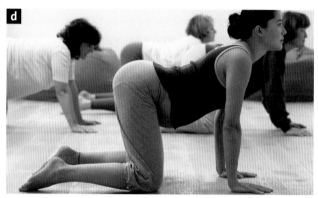

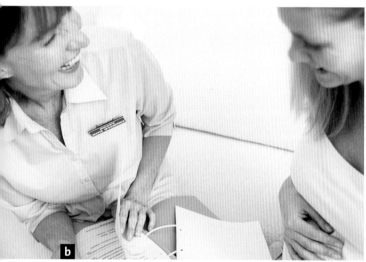

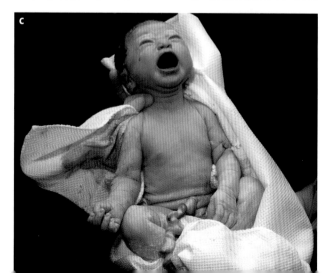

2 The incidence of Caesarean section in the UK was 23 per cent of labours in 2002. Nine per cent are pre-labour. How do these statistics for Caesarean section in the UK compare with your country?

3 Which is more common in your country – natural or managed labour? Do you think there is too much intervention in labour?

Listening

Taking details

1 Read this extract from a conversation between Mrs Canterbury and Dr Abboud. What are they talking about?

DOCTOR So, what can we do for you?

PATIENT Mmm, well, doctor, it's not really trouble, I think … I think [1]_____.

DOCTOR I see, and are you happy about that?

PATIENT Oh yes, [2]_____.

DOCTOR OK. Well, let's take some details. Can you remember when your last period was?

PATIENT Mmm, not exactly, but probably about six weeks ago.

DOCTOR So you think you've missed one?

PATIENT Yes. [3]_____.

DOCTOR Any other changes you've noticed?

PATIENT I do feel a bit sick most mornings, and my breasts feel a bit tender.

DOCTOR Right, if I give you a little bowl, can you just [4]_____ the toilet and bring back a sample for me?

2 What clues are there in the conversation to help you understand what is happening?

3 Complete the conversation using one of these phrases for each gap 1–4 in the conversation in **1**.

I'm as regular as clockwork
I'm expecting
I'm like a clock
I'm waiting for something
make a visit to
pop to
We've been practising for ages
We've been trying for ages

4 🎧 Listen and check your answers.

5 🎧 Who do you think says the phrases? Listen to the rest of the conversation. What do the phrases mean?

1 You're probably about four weeks gone.
2 We can usually get a clear picture.
3 I take it …
4 I do skip meals sometimes when I'm rushed.
5 There are certain things you need to steer clear of.
6 I haven't been on a binge for ages.

6 Check your answers with your partner.

7 Work in groups. Is the doctor very patient centred or very abrupt / businesslike? If necessary, how would you evaluate the doctor's manner and what improvements would you make?

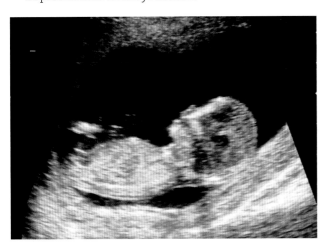

Signs and symptoms
Lay words and medical terms

1 What does the patient mean? Work in pairs. Translate the lay words into medical terms.

1 I haven't had a period for three months now.
2 I've been feeling sick in the morning. I keep throwing up, especially in the morning, and it's worrying me.
3 I haven't been for two days and it's the second time it's happened.
4 I think I've got piles.
5 I've come out in this rash on my tummy and arms. My mum says it will go when the baby's born, but I don't know.
6 I've been bringing up this horrible taste from my stomach.
7 I keep going to the toilet and passing water.
8 My back's killing me, especially at night.
9 I don't know what this brown patch is on my face.
10 I've got this tingling in the thumb and these two fingers.

2 Match each medial term with one of the patient's statements.

a haemorrhoids
b amenhorroea
c reflux oesophagitis and heartburn
d morning sickness
e constipation
f prurigo of pregnancy (PEP)
g urinary frequency
h paraesthesia
i chloasma
j lumbago

3 How would you reassure the patient in each case? Work in pairs. Take turns saying the statements and reassuring each other.

USEFUL EXPRESSIONS
It happens at this stage, but it'll … when the baby is born.
It's a good sign as it is associated with fewer foetal losses.

acknowledge (v) recognize / show

Speaking

Establishing rapport with patients is essential if you want them to cooperate with you. If you go straight into the medical aspect of the consultation without first acknowledging that the patient in front of you is a person, it can affect the history taking.

1 In *Listening*, the doctor starts the conversation with the safe subject of weather during which there are several very simple exchanges. For the 'safe' subjects in these pictures, decide how you would begin the consultation. What would you say?

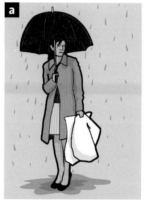
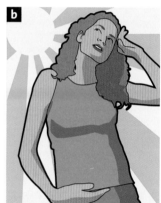
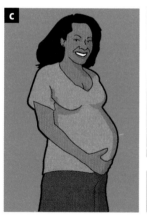
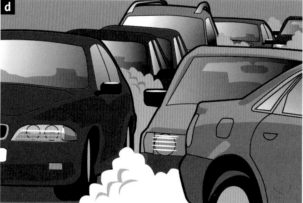
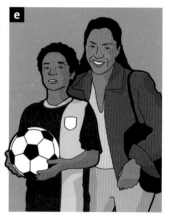

2 Which topics of conversation are better to avoid if you don't know the patient?

3 You may start the small talk or it may be started by the patient. How do you think the statements could be developed?

1 PATIENT It's still raining very hard out there.
2 PATIENT The weather's still awfully hot.
3 DOCTOR Hi. You look as if you are in a hurry today.
4 DOCTOR How has your work been recently / since I last saw you?
5 DOCTOR Hi. How are you? Fine? Good. I saw your husband with the children the other day. He was looking well after the op.
6 DOCTOR How's your mother since you brought her to see me last week?
7 DOCTOR [To child with mother] I see you're a football supporter. Have you been following the football on TV?
8 DOCTOR You're at university now. How's it all going?

4 Match these responses a–h to 1–8 in 3.
a It's wonderful. I ...
b Yes. I'm soaked through!
c Yes, but we mustn't complain. We might not have it for long.
d She's much better. Thank you for asking. It's really kind of you.
e Yes, I've been doing lots of different things this morning.
f Yes, I'm mad about football.
g It's been hectic, but fun. Thanks for asking.
h He's coming on very well. He's not looking forward to going back to work.

5 How long should the small talk last? How can you bring the small talk to an end?

6 Work in pairs. Take turns role-playing the beginning of a history from a patient and adding the phrases in 4. Develop it in your own way.

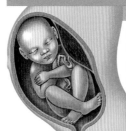

Foetus in breech position

ballot (v) push down as in pushing down an apple into water

placenta (n) the afterbirth

nucleus (n) main stress in the sentence

Vocabulary

Technical terms

1 Work in pairs. Complete the sentences by using one word from each list in each sentence.

A antepartum   birth   contractions   dilation
   lie   mother obstetric   placenta

B associated   cervix   defined   descends
   foetal   lifting longitudinal
   spontaneously

C dilated   fundus   gestation   haemorrhage
   pelvis   retained traction   ultrasound

1 The first stage of labour is the time from the onset of regular _____ until the _____ is fully _____.

2 After full _____ the head flexes further and _____ further into the _____.

3 A _____ not delivered in 30 minutes will probably not be expelled _____. The danger with a _____ placenta is haemorrhage.

4 The _____ usually reports absent _____ movements. There is no foetal movement (e.g. heartbeat) on _____.

5 A breech presentation is where the _____ on palpation is _____, no head is felt in the pelvis, and in the _____ there is a smooth round mass, which can be balloted.

6 _____ haemorrhage has been _____ as bleeding at >24 weeks' _____.

7 _____ of the posterior shoulder is aided by _____ the head upwards whilst maintaining _____.

8 Most _____ shock is _____ with severe _____.

2 Work in pairs. Choose one of the medical topics 1–8 in **1**. Prepare brief notes using your own knowledge and experience about the topic. Then swap pairs and use your notes to give a mini-presentation of two or three minutes about the topic to your partner.

3 Working with the same partner, choose a subject for your partner to talk about without preparation.

Pronunciation

Sentence nucleus

1 Find at least one word in *Vocabulary* for each stress pattern.

1 ●●●   4 ●●●●●
2 ●●●   5 ●●●●●
3 ●●●●

2 Identify the main stress or nucleus in the text in italics.

1 At vaginal hysterectomy, *the uterus is brought down through the vagina.*

2 *What happens is the womb is brought down through the vagina.*

3 *Pre-eclampsia is pregnancy-induced hypertension with proteinuria ± oedema.*

4 *It's a condition where the blood pressure is raised with protein in the urine and possibly swelling.*

5 *Normal labour is often heralded by a show.*

6 *When an induction is being planned,* the state of the cervix will be assessed.

7 *Ankle swelling is very common* when you're pregnant.

8 *It tends to worsen at night?* Well, if you use a firm mattress and wear flat shoes, it will help.

3 🎧 Listen and mark the nucleus and secondary stresses in the text in italics above. Check your answers with a partner.

4 Work in pairs. To help you feel the rhythm of the sentences, read only the words with secondary stress and the nucleus. Then read the full sentence. Check each other's responses.

5 Which of the sentences has more secondary stresses? Why is this so?

NCT (n) the National Childbirth Trust, a UK charity supporting parents

It's my job

1 Answer these questions before you read.

1 What happens in antenatal classes?
2 Are they a good use of resources in your opinion?
3 Who do you think should run such classes?

2 Now read the text. Are these statements true or false?

1 The antenatal course is restricted to pregnant women.
2 It is essential for trainers teaching in the name of the NCT to have the proper certification.
3 Antenatal classes are only held in hospitals.
4 The advice given is restricted to the pregnancy itself and the time immediately after pregnancy.
5 Pain relief is left to more specialist programmes run by midwives.

3 Work in groups. Are antenatal classes held in your country? If not, would they be useful? Give reasons. Who organizes / would organize the classes?

Mary Knox

I am Mary Knox, an NCT teacher of an antenatal course, which was set up to help prepare mothers for labour, their baby's birth, and early parenthood. This training is open to pregnant women, their partners, and their birth supporters. I have undergone a three-year training programme, which is unique in the world of childbirth education, leading to a diploma in Higher Education. In order to facilitate classes in the name of the NCT, teachers must hold a current licence to practise.

The antenatal programme I run is held in the evening for pregnant women and their partners (which may be the baby's father or another supporting person, such as a mother, sister, friend, or female partner). Some courses, however, may be held in a home or in a public venue and usually start at 30 weeks although sometimes 'early bird' classes are available earlier on in pregnancy. My present class covers

- what happens during labour and birth
- coping with labour (including information about pain relief)
- preparing for life with a new baby
- exercises to keep the mother fit during pregnancy and help her during labour
- how to care for a newborn baby

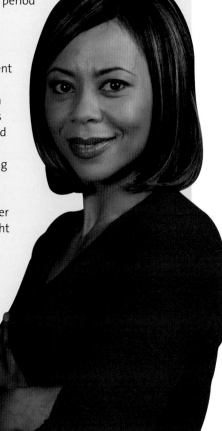

- looking after the mother's health during pregnancy (for example, nutrition and pelvic floor exercises) and after the birth
- the mother's feelings about pregnancy, birth, and the period after the birth.

The class also provides an opportunity to learn about and experiment with different birth positions and gives mothers the chance to learn about relaxation techniques (including massage skills and breathing techniques, for example). It's really gratifying giving pregnant women an opportunity to discuss the information available in order to make choices that are right for them. And it isn't just antenatal support we give. NCT classes create a support network because people make friends with others who are at a similar place in life.

the pill (n) the contraceptive pill

● **Language spot**

Giving advice and talking about expectation

1 Underline the correct modal verb in these sentences.

1 Are you saying that giving up smoking *should / can / must* improve our chances of having a baby?

2 *May / Must / Can* the epileptic drugs I'm taking affect the baby if I get pregnant?

3 Are there things I *can / ought to / may* be careful about during the first few weeks of pregnancy?

4 *Can't / Mustn't / Shouldn't* the baby be lying the other way round?

5 Do we *have to / ought to / need to* give up smoking and drinking then if we want to try for a baby?

6 *Can't / Must / Should* I see a specialist? Isn't it possible?

7 Do I *must / need to / should* have my baby in hospital? Can't I have it at home?

8 The doctor says I *can / must / should* rest for a couple of days. There is no alternative.

9 You think it *must / needs to* be to do with my blood pressure?

10 *Can't / Shouldn't / Mustn't* I just have one or two drinks during the pregnancy?

2 Work in pairs and categorize the statements in **1** as: *conclusion, persuasion, expectation, possibility, necessity, obligation, permission*. There may be more than one answer in each case, as when we speak, we convey several messages at one time.

3 Work in pairs and choose a question in **1** to ask your partner. Develop the conversation in your own way. Before you begin, look at *Grammar reference* on page 121.

4 Change partners and ask each other another question.

5 Imagine that you are a pregnant woman at an antenatal class. Think of questions to ask the antenatal teacher.

USEFUL EXPRESSIONS

Do you think I should ...?	*Are you saying I / we ...?*
Can't I (just) ... ?	*Do I / we have to ...?*
Do you think it must ...?	*Shouldn't I / we ...?*
Can I ...?	

>> Go to **Grammar reference** p 121

Speaking

1 Work in groups and discuss these scenarios.

● A 25-year-old patient who is epileptic, has a poor diet, and is taking the pill wants to become pregnant.

● A 25-year-old female whose partner smokes and drinks wants to have a baby. Both have a poor diet.

2 Make a list of the points you want to make and the questions you want to ask.

3 Choose one of the scenarios and take turns talking to the patient. The patient should try to use the questions in exercise **5** in *Language spot*.

USEFUL EXPRESSIONS FOR THE DOCTOR
If you want to ...
you can ...
you need to / it should ...
you are going to have to ...
[smoking] affects [egg production / sperm]

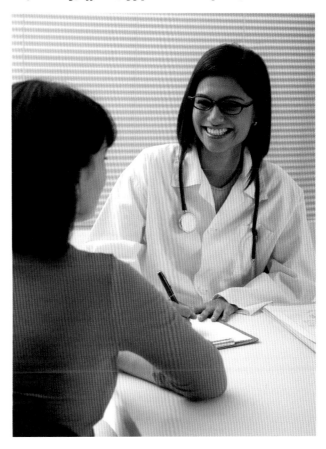

The pain is really your friend in labour. In these big transitions in life the pain is coming to help you. And that is such a different concept of pain; that pain is your friend instead of your enemy. It's the same as in big emotional problems. The pain actually helps you when you're grieving ...

– Well-known Dutch midwife, Beatrijs Smulders

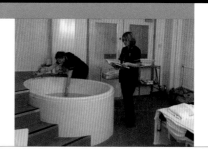

Reading

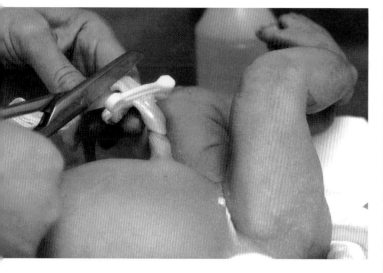

1 Before you start to read, use your own knowledge and make a list of the main points you would expect to see in an information leaflet for women about the third stage of labour.

2 Underline and number the words in the text that mean:
1 through
2 hold tightly
3 accelerate
4 triggered
5 previous
6 probability
7 throbbing

3 Use words from the passage to complete these sentences. In each case you will have to change the form of the word.
1 The third stage of labour ends with the
   _____ of the umbilical cord.
2 The _____ of bleeding does not necessarily rise in a natural third stage.
3 To quicken delivery a drug can be _____ into the patient's thigh.
4 When the placenta has _____ its task, the blood flow declines.
5 The _____ of the placenta in a managed third stage is caused by drug induced contraction.

Third stage of labour

Although, for convenience, health professionals divide labour into three stages, it is more useful to see labour as one continuous process with each preceding phase affecting what follows. The third stage of labour is the phase from the time when your baby fully emerges until the placenta is delivered. It is also the time when your baby adapts to life outside the womb.

There are two ways in which your placenta can be delivered. These are either a natural (physiological) third stage or a managed third stage.

A natural third stage means that no drugs are used to deliver the placenta. Instead it relies on the natural contraction of the uterus, stimulated by the surge of the hormone oxytocin at birth. This is the hormone that causes your uterus to contract and expel your placenta. A natural third stage does not increase the likelihood of severe bleeding if the labour has been normal and without epidural analgesia until then.

After your baby is born, the umbilical cord will be left intact. It is long enough so that you can hold your baby comfortably and begin the process of getting to know each other. As your baby adapts to life outside the womb the flow of blood from the placenta to your baby via the umbilical cord will decrease, as the role it has had during pregnancy comes to completion. The cord will only be cut and clamped when it has stopped pulsating. After a while you will begin to feel your uterus contract. At some stage you will feel your placenta in your vagina and push it out with a few small contractions. This stage can take anything from ten minutes to over an hour.

A managed third stage means that a drug (usually syntometrin or syntocinon) is given to speed up the delivery of the placenta. These drugs can cause nausea and vomiting and may raise the blood pressure in some women. They are given by injection into your thigh usually as your baby is being born or if requested, immediately afterwards. The main effect of this drug is an extra strong contraction. Your midwife will immediately clamp and cut your baby's cord so as to stop him receiving an abnormal surge of blood from the squeezed placenta. This strong contraction will have the effect of causing your placenta to peel away from the wall of your uterus. Other longer-lasting contractions will close the cervix, so your placenta will need to be delivered within about 7–8 minutes.

care plan (n) a system of care agreed with the patient

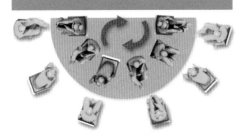

Speaking

1 Work in groups of three. Choose one of the topics. Imagine you are a patient and using your own experience, make notes about what you want to know from your doctor about the topic.

1 pre-eclampsia
2 anaemia in pregnancy
3 where to deliver
4 stillbirth
5 urinary frequency
6 hyperemesis gravidarum

2 Share your information with the rest of the class. Make some questions you think the patient might ask.

3 Divide into two groups of doctors and patients. Patients concerned with one of the topics 1–6 sit in a semicircle as per the diagram above. One doctor sits opposite each patient. The doctors have five minutes to speak to each patient and one minute for feedback.

4 At the end of the five minutes, the doctors move clockwise. After two or three patients, the doctors and patients switch roles and repeat the process.

Writing

Supporting opinions

1 Work in groups. Use your own experience to list the checks by weeks that a pregnant woman might need during pregnancy.

2 Work in pairs and imagine you are the patient. List the questions and concerns you would ask the doctor in this scenario.

> A young couple, Mr and Mrs Minton, are booking the antenatal care with your GP surgery. Mrs Minton is six weeks pregnant. She is primiparus and is in good health. They would prefer to have a home delivery. Answer their questions and address their concerns and then agree the care plan.

3 Take turns role-playing the scenario.

4 Work in groups. What type of essay are you being asked to write? Descriptive or argumentative?

> Delivery should only take place in a safe hospital environment. How far do you agree?

5 Brainstorm ideas for hospital and other types of delivery. Select three or four main ideas. Write a reason *(because)*, an example *(like / for example)*, an explanation *(If)*, additional information for each *(Moreover)*, a result *(And so / As a consequence / As a result)*. Then write about 250–300 words in answer to the question in **4**.

Checklist

Assess your progress in this unit. Tick (✓) the statements which are true.

- I can talk about pregnancy / giving birth
- I can use small talk
- I can speak smoothly and fluently
- I can understand lay language in obstetrics
- I can use modal verbs for negotiation

Key words

Nouns
afterbirth
breech
conclusion
expectation
lie
membranes
morning sickness
patch
period
pre-eclampsia
rapport
small talk
the Pill

Verbs
be expecting
rupture
try

Adjectives
antenatal
gone
longitudinal

Useful reference

Oxford Handbook of Clinical Specialties 8th edition, Collier and Longmore,
ISBN 978-0-19-922888-1

5 Psychiatry

Check up

1 Work in groups. Can you name these people?

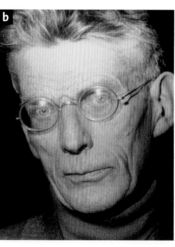
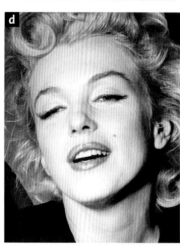
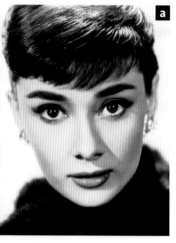
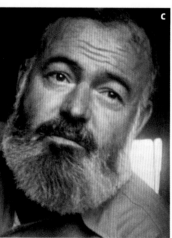

a Audrey Hepburn
b Samuel Becket
c Ernest Hemingway
d Marilyn Monroe

2 All of the above suffered from a depressive illness. Can famous people like these help remove the stigma of mental illness? How? Or do they confirm people's beliefs?

3 Are there any psychiatric illnesses in your country which are stigmatized? Are public attitudes changing or have they been the same for a long time?

Signs and symptoms

Psychiatric symptoms

1 Work in pairs. Can you identify the psychiatric symptoms below?

1 The emotional state prevailing in a patient at a particular moment and in response to a particular event or situation.

2 The loss of the ability to understand abstract concepts and metaphorical ideas leading to a strictly literal form of speech and inability to comprehend allusive language.

3 A normal and adaptive response to danger which is pathological if prolonged, severe, or out of keeping with the real threat of the external situation. There are two types: psychic and somatic.

4 Deliberately falsifying the symptoms of illness for a secondary gain (e.g. compensation, to avoid military service, to obtain an opiate prescription).

5 A sustained and unwarranted cheerfulness. It is associated with manic states and organic impairment.

6 The repetition of phrases or sentences spoken by the examiner. It occurs in schizophrenia and learning disability.

7 A severe and prolonged elevation of mood. It is a feature of manic illnesses.

8 A form of mood disorder initially characterized by elevated mood, insomnia, loss of appetite, increased libido, and grandiosity. More severe forms develop elation and grandiose delusions.

9 The subjective emotional state over a period of time.

2 Match these terms with 1–9 in 1.

a affect	d euphoria	g mood
b anxiety	e mania	h elation
c concrete thinking	f malingering	i echolalia

3 Write your own definition for one or more of these terms and compare them with other class members: *depressed mood, ataxia, clang association, bulimia, delusional mood, panic attack, somatization.*

4 In pairs, take turns giving definitions of the terms in 1–3. You can use: *Can you define ... for me?*

In this unit
- understanding basic definitions in psychiatry
- talking about affect and mood
- understanding and using lay terms
- using phrasal verbs
- understanding and pronouncing prepositions with verbs

5 In pairs, decide how to explain one or two of the terms in **3** to a patient. Then take it in turns role-playing the patient and doctor.

PATIENT
You can use: *Excuse me, but what does … mean?* Choose terms from the list that you have not prepared together to help prepare you for dealing with the unexpected.

DOCTOR
Use your own knowledge and experience to answer the patient's questions.

Listening 1

Mental state examination

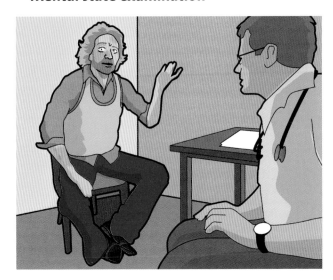

1 🎧 Listen to a doctor, Dr Vine, talking about the appearance, behaviour, and speech of one of the new patients as part of the mental state examination. Take notes under the three headings *appearance*, *behaviour*, and *speech*.

2 🎧 Compare your answers with a partner. Then listen again and check the details.

3 What other details would you want to know about for the examination under these headings: *mood, risk, anxiety, perception, thought, cognition, insight*? Use your own knowledge and experience.

4 What do you think the patient might say to indicate their mood, anxiety, or insight?

Patient care

1 Complete these patients' statements using a suitable word of your own.

1 I feel as if I'm on _____ of the world.

2 I'm always on _____, doctor, for no real reason. I'm a bundle of _____.

3 I just feel as if I'm weighed _____ by everything and everyone around me.

4 I get these _____ attacks when I try to get on buses or trains. I get pins and needles. I get out of breath and really tense as if something is going to happen.

5 I'm _____ out of my wits of leaving the flat. I don't know how I got here.

6 I do things like cleaning the house, again and again. I sometimes think I'm _____ my mind.

7 I'm feeling really _____ at the moment. I've been doing a lot of painting and I think I'm as good as Picasso, if not better.

8 I don't think I need much sleep. It seems such a _____ of time. I haven't been to bed for two days now and you see I'm OK.

9 Food? Oh, I have no _____ for preparing anything to eat or doing shopping.

2 Work in pairs. Categorize the statements according to whether you would associate them with anxiety or elation.

3 Work in groups. List and discuss other signs and symptoms you would expect in classic presentations of patients with anxiety or elation.

● **Language spot**
Phrasal verbs – separable and inseparable

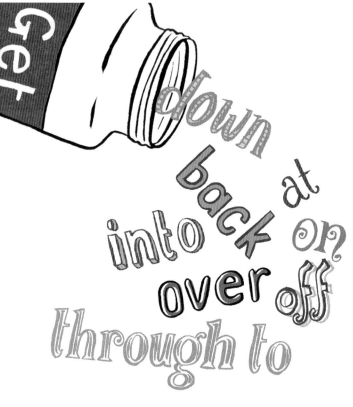

Get down at back into on over off through to

An understanding of phrasal verbs is another feature of colloquial English that will help you interpret and understand the patient.

EXAMPLES
Inseparable phrasal verb: I got into washing my hands again and again.
Separable phrasal verb: I couldn't fix it, which got me into a rage.

1 Work in pairs. Add the appropriate particle to each pair of sentences.

at	back	down	into
off	on	over	through to

1 a I feel as if everyone is getting _____ me all the time.
 b With so little information it's difficult to get _____ the diagnosis in this case.

2 a Sometimes work and the weather get me _____ .
 b Can you try and get some food _____ you today?

3 a My father got _____ his depression quite quickly.
 b He got the procedure _____ to the patient.

4 a I get _____ a violent temper quite easily these days at work and I know I shouldn't.
 b His depression got me _____ a bad mood too.

5 a It helps to try to talk about it so you can get it _____ your chest.
 b I find it very difficult to get _____ to sleep most nights.

6 a Everybody's getting _____ my nerves at the moment.
 b He gets _____ with everybody in the psychiatric ward.

7 a I've tried getting _____ Dr Jarvind but his bleeper appears to be faulty.
 b I've tried getting the importance of this message _____ him, but he's very resistant.

8 a He'll get _____ on his feet very quickly, so try not to worry.
 b When do you think I'll be able to get _____ to work?

2 Use these words to rewrite the relevant sentences in 1 where possible.

annoying (x2)	convincing (someone) of	contacting
depress me	eat some food	mastered
explained	release it	return

3 Write at least two sentences with the separable and inseparable phrasal verbs above about a patient you have treated. Work in pairs and describe the behaviour of the patient. Remember to maintain confidentiality.

>> Go to **Grammar reference** p 121

goldfish bowl (n) an arrangement where the audience for a role-play surrounds the performers so they can see both participants in the role-play

Speaking

1 Work in groups. Prepare questions you would ask a patient presenting either with anxiety or with elevated mood. Use the categories in the table below.

Anxiety	Elevated mood
Nature: *Would you say you were an anxious person?*	Mood: *How has your mood been lately? Do you find your mood is changeable at the moment?*
Severity:	Thoughts:
Precipitants:	Gifts / talents:
Impact on patient's life:	Sleep:
Situations / activities avoided:	Appetite:
Time spent on obsessional symptoms:	Concentration:

2 Work with a partner from another group. Do a role-play. Take turns taking a history from each other. The patient and the doctor should try to use the phrasal verbs in *Language spot*.

STUDENT A (PATIENT):
Do not tell the partner what your condition is. Decide on a name, age, and sex for the patient.

STUDENT B (DOCTOR):
Take a history from Student A. Bear in mind the Mental State examination above.

3 When you have finished, discuss any specific medical or language details that caused problems.

4 Now two volunteers perform the role-play again in 'the goldfish bowl'. Before the performance, turn to the speaking checklist on page 117 and, as a class, choose a criterion each to assess the performance. Take turns role-playing and giving feedback. The feedback should be constructive.

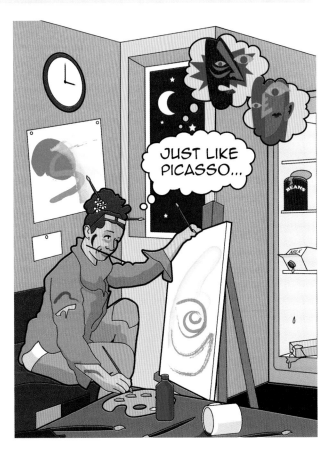

steeped in (v) immersed in

Reading

1 Below are the answers to questions about the reading text. Read the text then work in groups. Make questions beginning with *What*, using the words in brackets.

1 'vapours', 'hypochondria', or 'neuroses' (depressive disorder)
2 reduced functioning (other medical disciplines)
3 physiological (change / depression)
4 assumptions (affective disorders)
5 subjective symptoms (focus)
6 variable (neurotic or reactive depression)

2 Work as a whole class. Compare your questions with other groups and decide which group has the best question in each case.

3 Work as a whole class. Explain the answers using the information in the text.

The changing face of depression

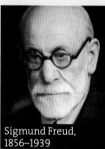

Sigmund Freud, 1856–1939

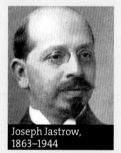

Joseph Jastrow, 1863–1944

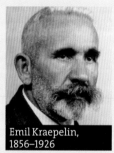

Emil Kraepelin, 1856–1926

OUR current ideas of what constitutes depression date from the mid-eighteenth century. Before that time, the old notion of melancholia, steeped in classical humoral theories (melancholia derived from the Greek *melaina* and *kole* 'black bile'), reflected intensity of idea. Sadness or low mood were not primary symptoms. The 'melancholic' symptoms we regard today as part of a depressive disorder would have been called 'vapours', 'hypochondria', or 'neuroses'. 'Depression', a term used to mean 'reduced functioning' in other medical disciplines, came to be associated with mental depression. It was adopted because it implied a 'physiological' change, and was defined as 'a condition characterized by a sinking of the spirits, lack of courage or initiative, and a tendency to gloomy thoughts.' (Jastrow 1901).

The concept was enlarged and legitimized by Kraepelin (1921) who used the term 'depressive states' in his description of the unitary concept of 'manic-depressive illness', encompassing melancholia simplex and gravis, stupor, fantastical melancholia, delirious melancholia, and involutional melancholia. A number of assumptions surrounded the affective disorders at that time: they involved primary pathology of affect, had stable psychopathology, had brain pathology, were periodic in nature, had a genetic basis, occurred in persons with certain personality traits, and were 'endogenous' (not related to precipitants).

In 1917, Freud published 'Mourning and Melancholia', influencing more than a generation in emphasizing cognitive and intra-psychic factors in the aetiology of depressive disorders, and shifting the focus of clinical descriptions from objective behavioural signs to subjective symptoms.

Over the intervening years, there has been much debate as to whether a 'biological' depression exists separate from a 'neurotic' type. Terminology has fluctuated around 'endogenous', 'vital', 'autonomous', 'endomorphic', and 'melancholic' depression, characterized by distinctive symptoms and signs, a genetic basis, and running an independent course unrelated to psychosocial factors. In contrast, 'neurotic' or 'reactive' depression could manifest in multiple forms, showed clear responsiveness to the environment, and ran a more variable course. Both ICD-10 and DSM −IV 'fudge' the issue somewhat by using severity specifiers (i.e. mild, moderate, severe) as well as 'symptom' specifiers (i.e. somatic symptoms, psychotic symptoms).

The advent of antidepressants introduced a further complication into the mix. Although Electroconvulsive Therapy (ECT) was widely accepted as a treatment for 'vital' depression, the idea of a drug treatment for 'reactive depressive disorders' ran counter to the received wisdom of the psychological basis to these conditions and the need for psychological treatment. ■

4 Discuss the contribution made to psychiatry by one or more of the people in the photos. Which was the most important development?

USEFUL EXPRESSIONS
The most important is (probably) ...
... has contributed the most / least to ...
If ... had not ...   Had he not ...

Baby blues: Up to ¾ of new mothers will experience a short-lived period of tearfulness and emotional lability starting two or three days after birth and lasting one to two days. This is common enough to be recognizable by midwifery staff and [may] require only reassurance and observation towards resolution.

– *Oxford Handbook of Psychiatry*

Vocabulary
Verbs with prepositions

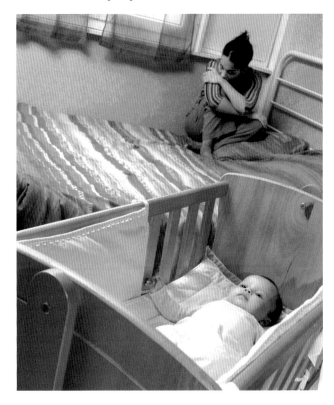

Each time you come across a verb, note the preposition that is used with it.

EXAMPLE
He was admitted to the psychiatric ward.

1 Look back at the reading passage and find the prepositions which are used with these verbs.

1 date	5 fluctuate
2 steep	6 manifest
3 derive	7 introduce
4 associate	

2 Work in groups. Add a word from each list below to complete sentences 1–8. You may have to change the form of the verb.

A	benefit	blame	come	cope	depend
	face	prescribe	think	worry	

B	about	for	from	from	of
	on	with	with	with	

1 I sometimes feel I can't _____ adequately _____ the baby as I am on my own with no support.

2 I never _____ myself unnecessarily _____ things that go wrong.

3 The baby _____ _____ me for everything and sometimes it all gets on top of me, but I look forward to every day.

4 I get down at times and sometimes feel a bit panicky and I don't know where it _____ _____.

5 My friend said you could _____ me _____ something to stop my mood fluctuations.

6 No, I can safely say I haven't _____ _____ harming myself or the baby at all.

7 I am _____ _____ so many things to do on my own that I don't know which way to turn at times.

8 I _____ _____ the baby a lot, especially about her health, but I wouldn't hurt her.

9 Would I _____ _____ seeing a counsellor, do you think?

3 Which sentences can you rewrite using these words? Are the prepositions the same in each case?

deal	fret	get something / anything out of
rely	reproach	stem / derive

Project

1 Search the web for the Edinburgh Postnatal Depression Scale (EPDS) or look in the *Oxford Handbook of Psychiatry*.

2 Work in groups. Discuss the significance of each of the ten items on the scale.

USEFUL EXPRESSIONS

associate with	*blame for*	*care for*
date from	*discuss with*	*distinguish*
from / between	*hint at*	*insist on*
react to	*relate to*	*stem from*
suffer from	*suspect of*	*think of*

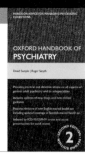

Always ask the patient about self harm or harming the baby.
– *Oxford Handbook of Psychiatry*

Pronunciation

Saying prepositions

1 🎧 Listen and complete the sentences below.

1 I can laugh _____.

2 It's difficult to distinguish one day _____.

3 Of course, I care _____.

4 I'm not trying to hint _____.

5 She insisted _____.

6 I sometimes blame myself _____.

7 The child depends _____.

2 🎧 Work in pairs. Check your answers. When you are sure the statements are correct, listen again.

3 What happens to the pronunciation of the preposition in each case? Can you copy the pronunciation? Practise repeating the sentences with your partner.

Speaking

1 Do a role-play.

1 Student A, go to page 114. Student B, take a history from Student A. Write notes as you listen and decide whether the patient is at risk or not.

2 Student B, go to page 116. Student A, take a history from Student B. Write notes as you listen and decide whether the patient is at risk or not.

2 Work in groups. Discuss the two cases. Give examples from your own or colleagues' experience, bearing in mind confidentiality. Try to use the verbs and prepositions in *Vocabulary* and *Project*.

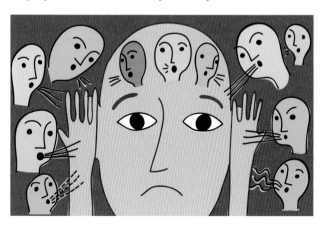

Listening 2

Asking about abnormal perceptions

1 🎧 Listen to a doctor asking a 30-year-old patient about abnormal perception. Complete the sentences.

DOCTOR   Now I want to ask you about some experiences which sometimes people have but find it difficult to talk about. 1_____. Is that OK?

PATIENT   Yeah.

DOCTOR   Have you ever had the sensation 2_____ or that the world had become unreal?

PATIENT   It's like ... I don't know how to explain it. It's ... I suppose it's like being in a play somehow. That maybe sounds as if I'm going mad.

DOCTOR   Have you ever had the experience of hearing noises or voices when 3_____?

PATIENT   Yes, sometimes.

DOCTOR   Is it OK 4_____?

PATIENT   Yeah, if you want.

DOCTOR   When did it happen?

PATIENT   The last time was a couple of days ago.

DOCTOR   Were 5_____?

PATIENT   Yeah, it was during the day.

DOCTOR   How often has it happened?

PATIENT   Recently only once or twice.

DOCTOR   And where did 6_____?

PATIENT   I don't know. From someone in the room.

2 Work in groups. Check your answers.

3 What other questions could the doctor ask about voices? What other questions can the doctor ask about taste or smell?

4 Do a role-play of the scenario above. Take turns taking a history.

5 Now perform the role-play in front of the class. Before doing so, turn to the speaking checklist on page 117 and, as a class, choose a criterion each to assess the performance. Take turns role-playing and giving constructive feedback.

Writing

Describing a chart

1 Work in groups. Describe the chart below. What is your reaction to the chart? Do you identify with the opinions of the medical groups?

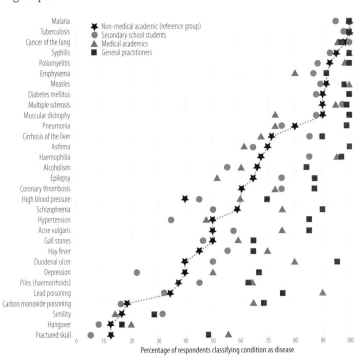

★ Non-medical academic (reference group)
● Secondary school students
▲ Medical academics
■ General practitioners

Percentage of respondents classifying condition as disease

2 Make a list of the most striking features of the chart and prepare a summary sentence or overview of all the data.

3 Describe the information in the chart in your own words. Write about 100–150 words. Then compare your description with a partner.

USEFUL EXPRESSIONS
While around 85 per cent of general practitioners think ..., only about 45 per cent of ...
Whereas ...
Whilst ...
a smaller proportion of / fewer secondary school students consider
More general practitioners than medical academics (approximately 90 per cent and 75 respectively) thought ...
believe / state / consider that
The percentage of... exceeded / surpassed / was greater than ...
a greater proportion of general practitioners (approximately 60%) than ... or ... state that

Key words

Nouns
abnormal perception
affect
anxiety
baby blues
elation
mania
mental state examination
mood

Verbs
benefit from
cope with
depend on
get at
get down
get on
get over
get through to
worry about

Adjectives
on edge
on top of the world

Useful reference

Oxford Handbook of Psychiatry 2nd edition, Semple et al, ISBN 978-0-19-923946-7

6 Geriatrics

Check up

1 Describe the pictures below.

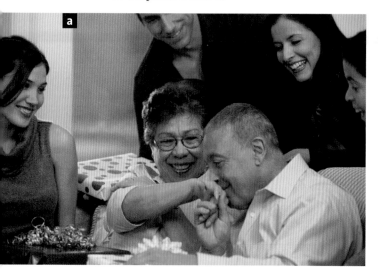

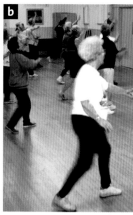

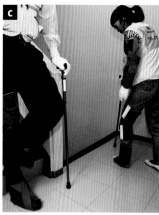

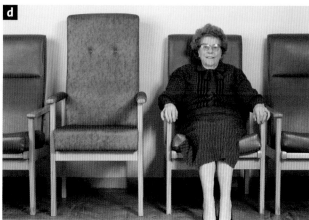

2 Work in groups. Discuss the questions.

1 What is the benefit of the young person wearing the training suit?

2 Why is it good to encourage elderly people to remain active?

3 Which picture reflects care in a home and which community care?

3 What is the proportion of elderly people in the UK and in your own country?

4 What is the difference between *handicap* and *impairment*? Find the answer in the WHO classification.

Listening 1

Picking up the thread of what is being said

It can be difficult to pick up the thread of conversations when people are speaking fast and when you come into them from outside once they have started.

1 🎧 Listen to the four conversation extracts and decide what each conversation is about.

2 🎧 Listen again, and when you think you have enough information to identify the topic of each conversation, ask for the conversation to be stopped.

1 _____   3 _____

2 _____   4 _____

3 What helped you work out the topic of the conversation?

4 What stopped you getting into the conversation immediately?

☐ not knowing the topic immediately
☐ the words
☐ colloquialisms
☐ the speed
☐ the voices themselves
☐ the short words
☐ listening to every word

5 Work in groups. Pool your answers. Then discuss what made it difficult or easy for you to understand the conversations and what strategies you used.

6 🎧 Listen to the conversations again. Do you understand them more?

In this unit
● understanding signs and symptoms
● supporting advice with purpose and reason
● *would, used to, get used to, be used to*
● talking about rehabilitation
● writing an essay with reasons

Signs and symptoms

Parkinson's and Alzheimer's

1 Look at the pictures. Decide which relates to Parkinson's disease and which to Alzheimer's disease.

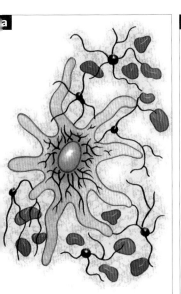

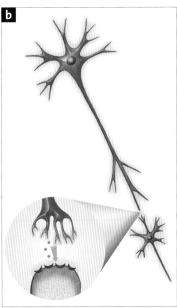

2 Work in pairs. What technical terms are being described? If you need help, check the list below.

1 He takes shuffling steps and he leans forward as if he is trying to keep up with his feet.
2 He has lost interest in everything.
3 His arms look as if he is carrying something heavy when he stretches them out.
4 He has lost all his sense of shame and keeps doing embarrassing things.
5 When he's relaxing, his hand shakes as if he's rolling pills between his finger and thumb.
6 It started off by his missing appointments when he used to be really punctual and getting the wrong end of the stick in conversations.
7 He just wanders off on his own and doesn't know where he is.
8 He takes his time starting off doing something.

anosognosia	apathy
bradykinesia	disinhibition
disorientation	rigidity
tremor	marche au petit pas / festinant gait

3 Which sentences in **2** relate to Parkinson's disease and which to Alzheimer's disease?

4 Work in pairs. Take turns eliciting a history from a woman whose husband presents with early signs of Parkinson's disease.

5 Explain to a son / daughter of a patient that their parent has Parkinson's disease. Point out the signs and symptoms of the disease. Refer them to the Parkinson's Disease Society and Age Concern. [Websites: www.parkinsons.org.uk and www.ageconcern.org.uk]

USEFUL EXPRESSIONS
What he's got is …
It's a condition where …
a mask-like expression – expressionless face
repetitive actions like typing
difficulty doing fine movements like picking things up
difficulty swallowing / dribbles
cog-wheeling – tremors imposed on rigidity
pill-rolling hands – worse at rest
morning stiffness
hesitates in starting movements

6 Work in pairs. Using the technical terms in **2** and your own experience, describe the signs and symptoms of a classic presentation of Parkinson's disease.

Project

Check the following sources for information on Alzheimer's disease.

● www.patient.co.uk
● the website for the Alzheimer's Disease Society
● the website for Age Concern
● the *Oxford Handbook of Geriatric Medicine*
● respite for the carer: www.carers.org

carer (n) someone who looks after a family member or friend on a long-term basis
respite (n) relief for a carer

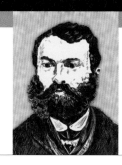

Dr. James Parkinson
1755–1824

• Language spot

would, used to, get used to, be used to

When we talk about repeated actions in the past which no longer exist we can use *used to* or *would*. They are generally interchangeable except *used to* can relate to continuous states like jobs which *would* cannot (unless it means a repeated action say on a particular day): *I used to work at St Mary's hospital on Thursdays / I would work at St Mary's hospital on Thursdays.*

Get used to means 'become accustomed to' and *be used to* means 'be accustomed to'.

1 Underline the correct alternative in each case below. In some cases both answers may be correct.

1 It's difficult *being / getting* used to the new regime of looking after my husband all day.
2 I *am used / am getting used* to doing everything for myself, so it's very distressing having someone like a carer do it.
3 He *would / got used to* take it into his head just to wander off for no reason whatsoever.
4 He *used to / would* work in the same hospital as me.
5 We *would spend / got used to spending* a lot of time in the library when we were undergraduates.
6 I can't *get / be* used to this night shift. On the geriatric ward, it's always busy.
7 He *used / 's used* to being turned every night in his bed, but he's getting too heavy for me to move.
8 I *didn't use to / wouldn't* spend much time doing exercise but now I wish I had.

2 Work in pairs. Each choose one thing you would do in the past, one thing you used to do, one thing you're getting used to now, and one thing you are used to. Explain to each other.

>> Go to **Grammar reference** p 122

Speaking

1 Work in groups. Collate the information that you collected about Alzheimer's disease for *Project*. Make a list of three to seven points that a husband or wife would be worried about regarding their spouse who may be suffering from the condition. Discuss the possible management of the case.

2 Work in groups of three with partners from another group. Take turns taking the history from each other about this scenario:

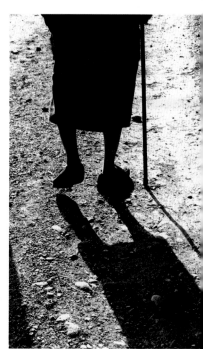

Mr Deacon presents with his wife, who has been suffering mood swings, forgetting things, and wandering off on her own. He compares what she used to be like and what they would do together. He is distressed by the experience. Take the history, explain the condition (after doing tests), and counsel the husband.

The doctor should explain what the diagnosis is after running some tests and offer a leaflet from the Alzheimer's Disease Society. Encourage Mr Deacon to think about respite for carers. Remember to be reassuring, sympathetic, and empathetic.

USEFUL EXPRESSIONS
This can't be easy for you (at all).
This must be really difficult for you, but ...
It's not easy coming to terms with this, but ...
It's difficult to come to terms with all this, but ...
Now and again, you'll need some time to yourself.
We are here to help you.

The positive features of dementia (Auntie Kathleen's syndrome) include wandering, aggression, flight of ideas, and logorrhoea:
'Not for her a listless, dull-eyed wordless decline; with her it is all rush, gabble, celerity. She had always been a talker, but now with her dementia unleashes torrents of speech ... one train of thought switching to another without signal or pause, rattling across points and through junctions at a rate no listener can follow ... Following the sense is like trying to track a particular ripple in a pelting torrent of talk.' – *Alan Bennett, Untold Stories.*

Reading

1 Find words or phrases with the same meaning as the following.

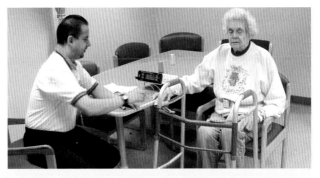

1 attacks or traumas
2 like or similar to
3 identify or describe
4 not strong
5 constant or reliable
6 involving the whole body
7 peripatetic

Rehabilitation

Rehabilitation is a process of care aimed at restoring or maximizing physical, mental, and social functioning. It can be used for acute reversible insults, e.g. sepsis; acute non-reversible or partially reversible insults, e.g. amputation, MI, and chronic or progressive conditions, e.g. Parkinson's disease. It involves both restoration of function and adaptation to reduced function depending on how much reversibility there is in the pathology. Rehabilitation is an active process done *by* the patient, not *to* him / her. It is hard work for the patient (akin to training for a marathon) – it is not convalescence (akin to a holiday in the sun).

Rehabilitation is the secret weapon of the geriatrician, poorly understood, and little respected by other clinicians. Many geriatricians feel it is what

defines their specialty and it can certainly be one of the most rewarding parts of the job. The 'black box' of rehabilitation contains a selection of non-evidence based, common sense interventions comprising:

- *positive attitude*. Good rehabilitationalists are optimists. This is partly because they believe all should be given a chance and partly because they have seen very frail and disabled older people do well. A positive attitude from the main team and other rehabilitation patients also improves the patients' expectations. Rehabilitation wards should harbour an enabling culture where the whole team encourages independence: patients dressed in their own clothes, with no catheter bags on show, and eating meals at a table with other patients.
- *multidisciplinary coordinated teamworking*. By sharing goals the

team can ensure they are consistent in their approach.

- *functionally-based treatment*, e.g. the haemoglobin level only matters if it is making the patient breathless while walking to the toilet.
- *individualized holistic outcome goals*. These incorporate social aspects which are often neglected. The team concentrates on handicap rather than impairment.

Specialized rehabilitation wards are not the only place for rehab. If the above considerations are in place then successful rehabilitation can take place in: acute wards, specialist wards (e.g. stroke units, orthopaedic wards), community hospitals, day hospitals, nursing and residential homes, and the patient's own home. The alternative sites often employ a roving rehabilitation team which may be used in hospital or the community.

2 Work in groups. In your own words explain the meaning of these phrases from the text and compare them with the rest of the class.

1 restoration of function and adaptation to reduced function
2 Rehabilitation is an active process done *by* the patient, not *to* him / her.
3 Rehabilitation is the secret weapon of the geriatrician
4 Rehabilitation wards should harbour an enabling culture
5 The team concentrates on handicap rather than impairment.

3 Work in groups. Describe the rehabilitation services that you have had experience of or are aware of. If none are available, what do you think could be done to help improve the quality of care for elderly patients in hospitals and at home?

One in ten persons is over the age of sixty. By 2050,
this proportion will have doubled to one in five.
– *Kofi Annan, former UN Secretary General*

Listening 2

Active listening

1 🎧 Listen to the recording of part of a conversation
between Dr Gonzalez and Mrs Day and decide what it
is about generally.

2 Map the consultation between the doctor and the
patient. Number the items 1–6 as they are mentioned
by the patient.

a _____ Medication

b _____ Pain puts her off exercise

c _____ Workmates upset her

d _____ Sleepless nights

e _____ Handicap

f _____ Lack of physiotherapy

3 Work in pairs. Answer the questions.

  1 Why doesn't the patient take the painkillers?
  2 Why is the concordance low?
  3 What handicap does the patient mention?
  4 What disability does the patient mention?
  5 How does the doctor seek to persuade the patient
    about the exercise?

4 🎧 Listen again and note two examples of active
listening by the doctor. What is the effect of this on the
patient?

5 Take turns role-playing the consultation between Dr
Gonzalez and Mrs Day. Decide how severe the pain is
and how cooperative the patient is. Remember to show
that you are listening actively at least twice during the
consultation.

● Language spot

Purpose and reason

During the
conversation between
Dr Gonzalez and Mrs
Day, the doctor tries
to encourage the
patient to do exercise
by explaining the
purpose for doing it:
*... to help improve your
strength and build up
your muscles, exercise
like swimming really
helps.*

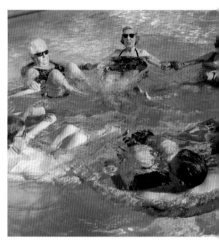

Supporting advice by giving reasons and the purpose
of rehabilitation treatment can help increase
concordance and hence independence in patients.

1 All of the phrases below contain purposes. Work in
groups. Decide which sentence endings match each
beginning.

  a We encourage people to have physiotherapy ...
  b We will visit your home ...
  c We are going to send you to rehabilitation ...
  d We are going to arrange a carer to come in once a
    day ...

  1 to get you ready for living on your own.
  2 to help with the pain.
  3 to see how you get on with doing things on your
    own.
  4 in order to assess how you can cope with cooking for
    yourself.
  5 to prevent falls.
  6 in order to rehearse the skills you need at home.
  7 to see if your home environment is suitable to
    return to.
  8 to ensure that it is feasible for you to leave hospital
    and that all possible problems and dangers have
    been minimized.
  9 to monitor how you are able to get around on your
    own with the walking frame.
  10 to help with washing in the morning.
  11 to improve coordination.

2 Work in pairs. Rewrite at least three of the sentences using the following constructions: *so that (we / you)* and *because*.

EXAMPLE
We encourage people to have physiotherapy because it reduces the pain. / so that we can help you with the pain.

3 Work in pairs. Take turns encouraging the patient, Mrs Day, to do some physiotherapy. Mrs Day can be as cooperative or uncooperative as you wish. Support what you say by giving reasons and stating purposes using the structures in this section.

>> Go to **Grammar reference** p 122

Vocabulary

Special equipment

1 Work in pairs. What are these items?

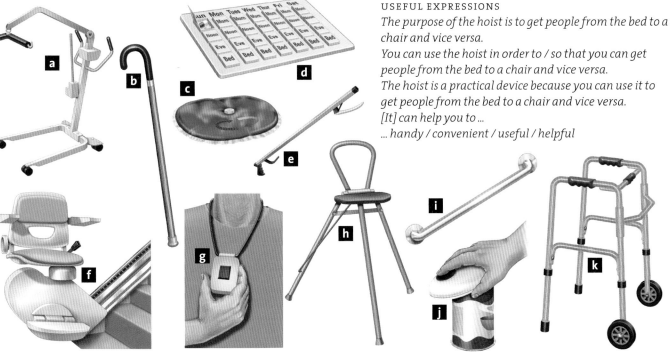

2 Work in pairs. Explain to each other the benefit of each of the items a–k. You may use the following sets of words to help you.

1. get people bed to chair and vice versa
2. dispense tablets patient safely
3. support walking
4. get up stairs
5. help ease pain
6. walk about house
7. call help problem fall
8. help go out street
9. pick something drop
10. open cans
11. lean / sit on when you get dizzy spells

3 Work in groups. Describe what aids are available for elderly people in your country.

4 Write sentences for items 1–11 using reasons and purposes.

USEFUL EXPRESSIONS
The purpose of the hoist is to get people from the bed to a chair and vice versa.
You can use the hoist in order to / so that you can get people from the bed to a chair and vice versa.
The hoist is a practical device because you can use it to get people from the bed to a chair and vice versa.
[It] can help you to ...
... handy / convenient / useful / helpful

a a hoist
b a walking stick
c a heat pack
d a Dossett box
e a helping hand
f a chair lift
g an alarm worn around the neck
h a perch
i a bar / rail (for the house)
j a special can opener
k a walking frame with wheels

rationing (n) limiting resources
irrespective (adv) regardless

FERTILITY RATE

In Europe 2.1 children per woman is considered to be the
population replacement level. These are national averages:

Ireland: 1.99   Sweden 1.75   Germany: 1.37   Greece: 1.29
France: 1.90   UK: 1.74   Italy: 1.33
Norway: 1.81   Netherlands: 1.73 Spain: 1.32

Source: *Eurostat – 2004 figures*

Speaking

1 Look at the scenario and prepare notes on your own.

> A 70-year-old patient, Mr / Mrs Lee, had been
> admitted for a hip replacement operation. The
> operation was successful and he / she wants to
> go home. However, he / she is not able to go home
> because he / she has no one to look after him / her
> and his / her home environment is not suitable.

2 Work in groups. Compare the information you
have gathered. Discuss the attitude of the patient
paying particular attention to the patient's feelings,
impairment, disability, and handicap.

3 Work in groups of three. Copy the checklist on
page 117. Two students role-play persuading the
patient to stay in the hospital and then to move to a
rehabilitation ward. Remember to indicate that you
are listening actively as the doctor. The third student
listens carefully to the conversation and writes down
as much information as possible.

USEFUL EXPRESSIONS
*It's better not ... because ... is not suitable because
... not practical / suitable convenient ... because ...
In order to / To make ... safer / more convenient / suitable ...
So that we can ...
Before we send you home we need to ... because*

4 The third student gives feedback about the
consultation. Discuss any inaccurate details and times
where it was difficult to follow the conversation.

5 Work on your own. Learning to speak impromptu
(without preparation) is a useful skill, but requires a
lot of practice. To help you start preparing, choose one
of the following topics. Using a stopwatch, spend two
minutes making notes to prepare a short talk on any
aspect of the items below relating to the elderly.

- pressure sores
- funny turns
- the flu
- hypothermia

6 Work in pairs. Place your notes so that your partner can
see them. Talk about the items you have noted for 3–5
minutes. Your partner should time the talk and allow
you to speak for no more than five minutes.

7 At the end your partner gives you feedback on how
closely you followed your notes.

Project

1 Work in groups. Look at the graph below taken from the
ONS (Office for National Statistics) or www.statistics.
gov.uk. What are the implications for health care of the
changing demographics? Are there similar projections
for your own country?

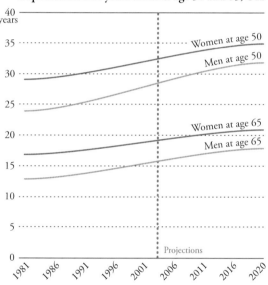

Expected further years of life at age 50 and 65, UK

2 Find projections for fertility rates on the ONS website
or Eurostat and / or check Eurostat for fertility rates in
the developed world.

Speaking

1 Divide into two groups: one group debate for and
one debate against the statement below. Spend ten
minutes preparing your arguments and then debate
the issue as a whole class.

> In health-care budgets there should be no rationing
> of resources and everyone should be treated equally,
> irrespective of age.

2 Appoint a student to make a list of the main arguments
for and against on the board or on a computer.

3 Choose another student to summarize the ideas at the
end. Take a class vote on the issue.

demographics (n) study of population and population changes

Writing

A short essay

1 Work in groups. Use these questions to help you analyse the essay topics a–c below.

1 Would you write about the topics in the same way or differently? How?
2 Are they the same type of essay?
3 Are they factual?
4 Does one require description only?
5 Do any of them require an evaluation where you state an opinion and support it by giving reasons or examples?
6 Can you use the factual information in one to support the reasons in another?

a How can governments overcome the problems associated with ageing populations?
b Explain how the changing demographics in the world are affecting health care provision.
c As the world's population ages, priority has to be given to the young and able bodied in allocating health care budgets. Rationing of health care is therefore inevitable. Do you agree?

2 Discuss the topics and prepare at least three ideas for each one. Each group should then present their ideas to the whole class.

3 For topic c, which adjective best sums up your attitude to the topic?

acceptable	flawed	immoral	indefensible
objectionable	offensive	unacceptable	unethical
unjustifiable	unreasonable	untenable	watertight
wrong			

4 Write about 200 words about topic c.

USEFUL FRAMES
[The main reason is that] [...] is unethical because ...
For example, if we look at ... Moreover, the purpose of health care is to ... Therefore, ...

USEFUL EXPRESSIONS
The main reason is
Another reason is
Governments need to / should
Take, for example,
If we take, for example, where ...
... can(not) be justified (by) ... (because)

Key words

Adjectives
ageing
impromptu
shuffling

Nouns
anosognosia
apathy
bradykinesia
disability
disinhibition
evaluation
gait
handicap
impairment
marche à petit pas
rehabilitation
rigidity
thread
tremor

Verbs
analyse
pick up

Useful reference

Oxford Handbook of Geriatric Medicine, Bowker et al, ISBN 978-019-853029-9

Reading bank

1 Triage

1 Work in pairs. Explain what you understand by the term *triage*. Compare your answer with other students.

2 Read the text. Complete the sentences below using words from the text. You may have to change the form of the word.

1 Triage is a system where patients are prioritized for treatment to make sure those whose problems are most _____ are seen immediately.

2 The purpose of the triage process is to put patients into _____ according to their need medically and the resources available in the department.

3 Patients who need to be seen instantly are indicated in _____ .

4 If patients do not need to be seen within two hours, they are categorized as _____ on the scale with the colour _____ .

3 Answer the following questions.
1 What qualities of a triage nurse are mentioned?
2 What examples of instant treatment are mentioned for all patients?
3 How long does triage normally take?
4 Why is triage described as a dynamic process?
5 What category change is quoted to illustrate the dynamic process, standard to very urgent or very urgent to standard?

4 Work in pairs. Complete the text in the last paragraph, using the words below:

uncomplaining	urgent	aware
non-urgent	inordinately	

Triage

The nature of triage of Emergency department work means that some sorting system is required to ensure that patients with the most immediately life-threatening conditions are seen first. A triage process aims to categorize patients based on their medical need and the available departmental resources. The most commonly used process in the UK is the National Triage Scale where the scale of urgency is indicated by a colour for ease of reference.

National Triage Scale	Colour	Time to be seen by doctor
1 Immediate	Red	Immediately
2 Very urgent	Orange	Within 5-10 minutes
3 Urgent	Yellow	Within 1 hour
4 Standard	Green	Within 2 hours
5 Non-urgent	Blue	Within 4 hours

As soon as a patient arrives in the emergency department he or she should be assessed by a dedicated triage nurse (a senior, experienced individual with considerable common sense). This nurse should provide any immediate intervention needed (eg elevating injured limbs, applying ice packs or splints, and giving analgesia) and initiate investigations to speed the patient's journey through the department (eg ordering appropriate X-rays). Patients should not have to wait to be triaged. It is a brief assessment which should take no more than a few minutes.

Three points require emphasis:

Triage is a dynamic process. The urgency (and hence the triage category) with which a patient requires to be seen may change with time. For example, a middle-aged man who hobbles in with an inversion ankle injury is likely to be placed in triage category 4 (green). If in the waiting room he becomes pale, sweaty and complains of chest discomfort, he would require prompt re-triage into category 2 (orange).

Placement in a triage category does not imply a diagnosis, nor even the lethality of a condition (eg an elderly patient with colicky abdominal discomfort, vomiting, and absolute constipation would normally be placed in category 3 (yellow) and a possible diagnosis would be bowel obstruction). The cause may be a neoplasm which has already metastasized and is hence likely to be ultimately fatal.

Triage has its own problems. In particular, patients in _____ categories may wait _____ long periods of time, whilst patients who have presented later, but with conditions perceived to be more _____ , are seen before them. Patients need to be _____ of this and to be informed of likely waiting times. _____ elderly patients can often be poorly served by the process.

2 Preventing injuries

1 Work in pairs. Are accidents at work easily preventable? Give reasons and examples from the field of medicine.

2 Read the text. In pairs, find verbs that mean the same as the following. The verbs in the text will be in different forms.

1 put
2 avert
3 find / isolate
4 hit
5 suggest
6 disconnect
7 connect
8 get down
9 check
10 declare

3 Work in pairs. All of the statements below are false. Find the evidence in the text.

1 The Summary mentions the recommendations as regards health and safety in all work situations.
2 Three main causes of injury by excavators or backhoe loaders have been identified from the data.
3 Cave-ins are the only other main factors mentioned as leading to death.
4 In Case study 1, the victim was rushed to hospital.
5 In Case study 2, the victim was climbing a building when the accident happened.

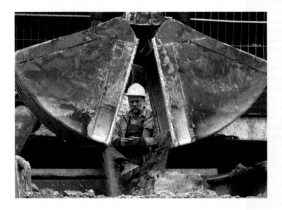

Preventing injuries when working with hydraulic excavators and backhoe loaders

Summary

Workers who operate or work near hydraulic excavators and backhoe loaders are at risk of being struck by the machine or its components or by excavator buckets that detach from the excavator stick. The National Institute for Occupational Safety and Health (NIOSH) recommends that injuries and deaths be prevented through training, proper installation and maintenance, work practices, and personal protective equipment.

Description of exposure

A NIOSH review of the Bureau of Labour Statistics (BLS) Census of Fatal Occupational Injuries (CFOI) data identified 346 deaths associated with excavators or backhoe loaders during 1992–2000 [NIOSH 2002]. Review of these data and of NIOSH Fatality Assessment and Control Evaluation (FACE) cases [NIOSH 2000, 2001] suggests two common causes of injury: (1) being struck by the moving machine, swinging booms, or other machine components; or (2) being struck by quick-disconnect excavator buckets that unexpectedly detach from the excavator stick. Other leading causes of fatalities are rollovers, electrocutions, and slides into trenches after cave-ins.

Case study 1

A 28-year-old labourer died after he was struck by the bucket of a hydraulic excavator. The victim, a co-worker, and the operator were using an excavator equipped with a quick-disconnect bucket to load concrete manhole sections onto a truck. The victim was on the ground to connect the manhole sections to the excavator while the co-worker was on the truck to disconnect the sections after they had been loaded on the truck. The operator had positioned the excavator bucket near a manhole section while the victim attached a three-legged bridle to the manhole section for lifting. The bucket disconnected from the excavator stick (Figure 1) and struck the victim. He was pronounced dead at the scene [NIOSH 2001].

Case study 2

A 32-year-old construction labourer died after being struck in the head by a backhoe bucket. The victim was part of a two-man crew clearing earth away from the foundation footing of a house. The backhoe operator began digging an approximately 60 cm-wide by 60 cm-deep excavation around the foundation while the victim used a hand shovel to remove extra earth after the backhoe had passed through. The amount of footing protruding was decreasing. The operator lowered the backhoe's bucket to rest on a pile of earth approximately 8 ft from the victim; he then dismounted from the backhoe to inspect the trench. When the operator returned to the machine and stepped over the tyre to sit down, he inadvertently contacted the boom swing control, swinging the boom toward the victim standing in the trench. The boom struck the victim, pinning him against the house. He was pronounced dead at the scene [NIOSH 2000].

3 How dangerous is skiing?

1 Work in groups. Read the text, then match the paragraph headings below to the paragraphs A–E.

1 Are there too many people on the slopes?
2 Why are boarders and skiers in conflict?
3 So has skiing become very high-risk?
4 Are helmets the answer?
5 How hard is it to avoid skiing into someone?

2 Work in pairs. Use no more than three words from the text to complete each sentence.

1 According to research, skiing is less dangerous than playing a

_____ .

2 A crucial factor in becoming proficient in mountain skiing is

_____ .

3 Sometimes more ski slopes cannot be created because the

_____

of the land makes access to the slopes difficult.

4 Wearing a helmet increases the chance of people taking more

_____ .

5 Snowboarders are more exposed to possible _____ than skiers.

3 Work in groups. Should greater controls be introduced into sports to reduce the risk of injuries? Give reasons. Do controls for children reduce the enjoyment of sports? Does such risk averse control reduce children's development?

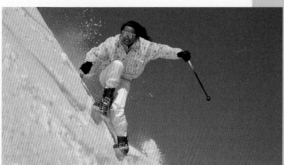

The Big Question: Is skiing now so dangerous that speed limits should be imposed?

A It's all relative. There are no overall statistics on skiing injuries across the world, but individual studies suggest people's fears may be exaggerated. The Aviemore-based sports injury research facility ski-injury.com reports that only 1.74 alpine skiers per 1,000 will sustain an injury, so statistically it's safer than a game of football. In addition, only ten per cent of skiing injuries are caused through collisions. Most are caused by the skier either falling over or skiing into a tree or other object.

B Most accidents happen when people get tired, so the last run of the day is traditionally quite busy for emergency services. Even on the widest of skiing motorways, it is very possible to collide with another skier – spatial awareness is a key element to mastering alpine skiing. Certain resorts have 'pinch points' where a lot of traffic passes at the end of the day as people funnel down the mountain, and when boy racers lose patience and decide to queue-jump the orderly procession, people get knocked over.

C According to the Ski Club of Great Britain (SCGB), since 2001 the total snow sports travel market has increased by 23 per cent. That's nearly a quarter additional skiers using, in many cases, the same acreage of space. In many resorts, it is simply not possible to create more runs, as the land is often privately owned, belongs to protected national parks, or doesn't have the right topography to allow for easy access. Last season was a bumper year for skiers, with superb snow conditions across much of Europe and North America; to this end, some 1.35m travellers headed for the slopes.

D At the moment, there is no law on wearing a 'lid' on the slopes, but the SCGB recommends that children under thirteen wear one and leaves it up to the discretion of the individual from there on up. The helmet has become a fashion statement in recent years and is used by all professional freeriders and boarders, who spend their entire time jumping out of helicopters in the most remote ski fields in the world. By wearing one you can associate with this romanticism, even if you never stray from the piste, so this is a force for good. Having said that, the helmet does lead some people to think that they can take more risks as they are protected, so it leads to a false sense of security.

E Why are boarders and skiers such a combustible mix? This could be the subject of its own Big Question, but generally the two approach the mountain in two entirely different ways. A skier has to have attained a level of proficiency in order to tackle the slopes that a snowboarder will not have had to. In short, there are more 'bad' amateur snowboarders who take to the slopes than there are 'bad' amateur skiers. Snowboards – which attract the younger and possibly more reckless thrill-seeker – simply don't have the same control and grip as two independently controlled skis, and without a set of poles, a boarder who wants a rest simply sits down, which makes them less visible and therefore more vulnerable to potential collisions.

4 Fathers and pregnancy

1 Work in pairs. Is it common for fathers to be present at the birth of their children in your country? Why / Why not? What do you think of the idea? Give reasons.

2 Read the text. In pairs, match the names 1–7 to the list of items a–g.

  1 Kiernan and Smith, 2003
  2 Scott et al, 2001
  3 Wolfberg et al, 2004
  4 Venners et al, 2005
  5 McLeod et al, 2002
  6 Chang et al, 2006
  7 Penn and Owen, 2002

  a showed that mother's smoking is related to a father's smoking.
  b stated that childhood leukaemia is connected with fathers' smoking.
  c showed that prenatal information for fathers has an effect on mothers' breastfeeding habits.
  d showed that the majority of fathers are present at their child's birth.
  e stated that early pregnancy loss is greater when fathers smoke.
  f stated various studies show fathers have an effect on mothers' breastfeeding decisions.
  g stated that mothers stop breastfeeding early when fathers smoke.

3 Work in pairs. Has the text changed your answers to the questions in 1 above? Given reasons.

The role fathers play in supporting their pregnant partners

A social revolution unimaginable 50 years ago is taking place every day in the UK's maternity units – a huge majority of fathers now attend the birth of their children.

One analysis of national statistics (Kiernan and Smith, 2003) puts the overall percentage at 86%. This figure rose to 93% for fathers living with their child's mother (more than four out of five couples are living together at the time of the birth). Among the couples not living together at that time, but still having a positive relationship with each other (one in ten couples), 64% of fathers were at the birth. Even where fathers were described as 'not in a relationship' with the mothers (one couple in twenty), 10% of the fathers were present at the birth (Kiernan and Smith, 2003).

There is a public debate about the importance of fathers, with politicians on both sides of the Atlantic – notably Barack Obama and David Cameron – focusing on the threats posed by absent or disengaged dads, especially those in minority ethnic communities. And yet the very services that are best positioned to kick-start a more positive, engaged relationship between fathers and the State – maternity services – only ask two formal questions about fathers: if there are any genetic abnormalities on their side of the family and whether they are violent.

This cannot be the best we can do, given what we know about the significant positive impacts that engaging with fathers can have on the health of mother and baby.

Take breastfeeding – a number of studies have found that fathers' behaviour and attitudes influence mothers' decisions to initiate and / or sustain breastfeeding (Scott et al, 2001). Wolfberg et al (2004) conducted a small randomized controlled trial that consisted of a two-hour prenatal intervention with fathers, where they were given infant care information and encouraged to advocate breastfeeding and assist their partner. It resulted in a 74% breastfeeding initiation among women whose partners had attended the class, compared with 41% for the control group.

Fathers' smoking is associated with increased risk of early pregnancy loss (Venners et al, 2005), early cessation of breastfeeding (correlation independent of maternal smoking) (McLeod et al, 2002), and childhood leukaemia (Chang et al, 2006). It is also the biggest predictor of the mother's smoking status (Penn and Owen, 2002), and mothers who stop smoking are consistently associated with fathers' provision of support and quitting themselves (McBride et al, 2004). Research suggests that becoming a father can be a 'significant life event' that increases receptiveness to smoking cessation influences, and that providing expectant and new fathers with targeted information about the effects of passive smoking on babies can help them quit (Burgess, 2007). Does your maternity service focus on fathers' and mothers' smoking behaviour at this time?

5 OCD

1 Work in groups. What do you know about the causes of obsessive compulsive disorder (OCD)? Have you treated any patients with OCD? Describe the presentation of the disorder.

2 Read the text. Answer the questions *yes* or *no*.

1 Has a link between OCD and the structure of the brain in sufferers and their near relatives been established?

2 Does a sizeable proportion of the population have OCD?

3 Is the fear of dirt one of the obsessions suffered by patients with OCD?

4 Is OCD inherited?

5 Were only brains of healthy parents of OCD sufferers tested in the Cambridge research?

6 Was the completion of a questionnaire on the computer by the patients part of the research?

7 Did the near relatives of OCD sufferers do better than the control group?

3 Give the correct information for the questions in **2** where the answer was no.

4 Work in pairs. As quickly as you can, find adjectives in the text which have the same meaning as:

1 unconnected
2 domestic
3 common
4 characteristic
5 recurring
6 comparable
7 enhanced
8 causative
9 fundamental.

Brain pattern associated with genetic risk of OCD

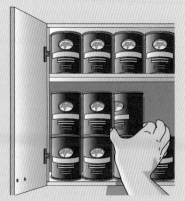

Cambridge researchers have discovered that individuals with obsessive compulsive disorder (OCD) and their close family members have distinctive patterns in their brain structure. This is the first time that scientists have associated an anatomical trait with familial risk for the disorder.

These new findings, recently reported in the journal *Brain*, could help predict whether individuals are at risk of developing OCD and lead to more accurate diagnosis of the disorder.

Obsessive compulsive disorder is a prevalent illness that affects 2–3% of the population. OCD patients suffer from obsessions (unwanted, recurrent thoughts, concerns with themes of contamination and 'germs', the need to check household items in case of fire or burglary, the symmetrical order of objects, or fears of harming oneself or others) as well as compulsions (repetitive behaviours related to the obsessions such as washing and carrying out household safety checks). These symptoms can consume the patient's life, causing severe distress, alienation, and anxiety.

OCD is known to run in families. However, the complex set of genes underlying this inheritability and exactly how genes contribute to the illness are unknown. Such genes may pose a risk for OCD by influencing brain structure (e.g. the amount and location of grey matter in the brain) which in turn may impact upon an individual's ability to perform mental tasks.

In order to explore this idea, the researchers used cognitive and brain measures to determine whether there are biological markers of genetic risk for developing OCD. Using magnetic resonance imaging (MRI), the Cambridge researchers captured pictures of OCD patients' brains, as well as those of healthy close relatives (a sibling, parent, or child) and a group of unrelated healthy people.

Participants also completed a computerized test that involved pressing a left or right button as quickly as possible when arrows appeared. When a beep noise sounded, volunteers had to attempt to stop their responses. This task objectively measured the ability to stop repetitive behaviours.

Both OCD patients and their close relatives fared worse on the computer task than the control group. This was associated with decreases of grey matter in brain regions important in suppressing responses and habits.

Lara Menzies, in the Brain Mapping Unit at the University of Cambridge, explains, 'Impaired brain function in the areas of the brain associated with stopping motor responses may contribute to the compulsive and repetitive behaviours that are characteristic of OCD. These brain changes appear to run in families and may represent a genetic risk factor for developing the condition. The current diagnosis of OCD available to psychiatrists is subjective and therefore knowledge of the underlying causes may lead to better diagnosis and ultimately improved clinical treatments.

'However, we have a long way to go to identify the genes contributing to the distinctive brain structure found in OCD patients and their relatives. We also need to identify other contributing factors for OCD, to understand why close relatives that share similar brain structures don't always develop the disorder.'

6 Nifty after fifty

1 Work in groups. The text is about gyms for elderly people or 'seniors'. Why do you think gyms like this are beginning to be opened? Are such gyms common in your country? If not, would they be popular? Give examples and reasons.

2 Read the text. As quickly as you can, find words and phrases in the text which have the same meaning as the following:

1 weakening
2 appearing
3 do exercise
4 hectic
5 frightened
6 focusing on
7 agile
8 expanded
9 available to spend
10 attracts.

3 Find the person or organization that gave the information below. You may use each name more than once.

1 there were not many gyms for elderly people at the end of the last century
2 the number of people joining health clubs is increasing
3 older people are frightened by the music and the very fit people in gyms
4 the number of elderly people is increasing
5 the queries about gyms for older people are not restricted to one area

4 Work in groups. What is your opinion about the development of gyms for senior / elderly people? Give reasons and examples.

More seniors-only fitness centers popping up

NEW YORK – Marshall Kahn attends a gym with yoga, tai chi and Pilates classes, weight training, and treadmills. It also has a driving simulator, where members can keep their skills from deteriorating.

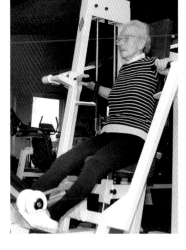

The gym, Nifty After Fifty, is one of many fitness centers popping up around the country aimed at serving older clients. 'I'm 80, my wife is 48. So I have to stay fit,' said Kahn, who signed up at one of the company's four Los Angeles locations earlier this year and pays about $50 per month to work out three times a week. 'I joined a gym about three or four years ago, and I didn't like it at my age – it was young, noisy, and frenetic. They were doing all these crazy things I couldn't participate in. Here, I'm not intimidated. I'm more inclined to go.'

When it comes to designing a gym, it's not all about attracting the hard bodies any more, and when it comes to senior fitness, there's more out there than water aerobics. As more of America's baby boomers start entering their 60s, more startup gyms are homing in on a more mature market.

Gentler atmosphere

'As we get older, we're sort of intimidated about going into a 25,000 square-foot gym with rock music and people in tight leotards and muscles bulging from every aspect of their T-shirts,' said 74-year-old Sheldon Zinberg, who opened Nifty After Fifty last year.

Nifty After Fifty plays softer music than the typical gym, and uses smooth, air pressure-driven equipment for strength training as opposed to your typical metal weights. So does Healthfit, a club based in Needham, Mass., where paintings adorn the walls and the average client is over 50. FitWright – a club that opened last fall in Dedham, Mass., which has seen particular interest recently from people in their 60s and 70s – offers a special 'gentle yoga' class for its less limber members.

'I think more than half the calls I get, and there's no regionality to this, are about doing a senior-only health club,' said John Atwood, who runs Healthfit and the consulting firm Club Management Group, which advises small or mid-size clubs. 'There was very little of this in the 90s.'

The business potential is huge, and expanding. Club 50, a fitness chain for the over-40 crowd that has mushroomed to more than 40 franchises since it began in 2003, points out that seniors control more than 70 per cent of the country's disposable income.

And the oldest of the baby boomers, born between 1946 and 1964, started turning 60 last year. In less than 25 years, there will be more than 71 million 65-year-olds, twice as many as there were in 2000, according to the National Association of Area Agencies on Ageing.

The US health club industry pulls in about $16 billion in annual revenue, according to data from the International Health, Racquet & Sportsclub Association. Over the last twenty years, the number of people with club memberships has more than doubled and the number of clubs has nearly tripled, IHRSA's data show.

7 Roman face cream

1 Work in pairs. Look at the title and skim the text. What is the text about?

2 Read the text. Replace the text in bold below with words and phrases from the text.

1 A small tin which was a gift to Roman gods was **found** recently.
2 The contents of the tin were found to be **intact**.
3 The experts were **very surprised by the contents of the tin**.
4 Creams from the Roman period **usually perish**.
5 **An analysis will take place shortly** to ascertain the purpose of the cream.
6 Historians **suggested the gift was possibly donated** by a wealthy Briton rather than a Roman.
7 The archaeological site will **become a building complex**.

3 Make questions for the information in each statement in **2**. Use *who* and *what*.

1 uncover lately?
2 contents tin?
3 reaction when open tin?
4 happen Roman cream?
5 perform in the near future?
6 historians propose who made the donation?
7 happen to the archaeological site?

4 Work in groups. Do you think cosmetics are used more now than in the past? Does advertising persuade people to buy cosmetics unnecessarily?

Roman face cream found at London temple site

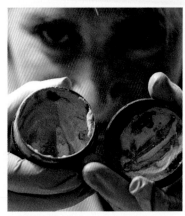

A SMALL TIN can hidden in a ditch at a Roman temple as an offering to the gods was opened for the first time in nearly 2,000 years yesterday to reveal what appeared to be smelly old face cream.

The sulphurous-smelling ointment was discovered to be complete with a genuine fingerprint of a Roman subject on the lid.

The sealed container – the size of a tin of sweetcorn – was found more than a week ago during an archaeological dig at the first temple complex of its kind discovered in London.

The can – which museum staff suspected might have contained gold, beads, or a small statue – had been buried in an old drain at the site in Southwark, south London.

It was unsealed yesterday at the Museum of London. After Liz Barham, a conservator, carefully unwrapped the container and unscrewed the lid, experts said they were stunned to discover what was inside.

Gary Brown, managing director of Pre-Construct Archaeology, which discovered the pot, said: 'I don't think we could have expected that it would be so full, or that it would be some kind of cosmetic, moisturizing cream or whatever it is. Clearly Roman creams of any type, paint or cosmetic, do not normally survive ... it's pretty exceptional.'

Tests to be carried out soon will reveal if the ointment is face cream, a form of face paint daubed for religious services, or something completely different.

Nansi Rosenberg, senior archaeological consultant on the project, said: 'We know they [Romans] were very keen on appearance, used earlobe scrapers and tweezers, and there are a lot of Roman baths around.'

Historians said that the offering may well have been made by a member of the emerging British 'bourgeoisie' who had got wealthy through the rise of the Roman Empire.

The temple site was built at a point where the roads to London from Chichester and Dover met – suggesting a stopping point on one side of London. It has provided rare evidence of organized religion in the capital.

The complex, which dates from the middle of the second century AD, is believed to have been a religious meeting point from when native Celtic and Roman cultures had become entwined. The remnants of two small square temples were found, along with a possible guesthouse, an area for outdoor gatherings, plinths for statutes, and a column base. Items of historical importance have been removed and the site will now be converted to homes, offices, and shops.

8 Training for surgeons

1 Work in groups. Do you think that it is difficult for surgeons to keep up with modern surgical techniques? Give reasons. How do you keep up to date?

2 Work in pairs. Underline the phrases in the text which you can replace with the following:

1 do not have any sensation of touch
2 a standard
3 not an objective appraisal
4 it is not practical
5 has had an impact on current procedures
6 is not wholly effective
7 is inadequate

3 Scan the text for the answers to the questions as quickly as possible. Time yourself and compare your time with other students.

1 What has happened swiftly in the recent past?
2 Which downsides of Chmarra's training system are mentioned?
3 How many training methods are used for minimally invasive surgery? What are they?
4 What criticisms are voiced of the training methods?
5 Does Chmarra's device work?

4 Work in groups. How do you prefer to learn new techniques and procedures, surgical or otherwise? Give examples.

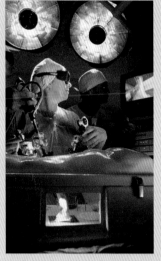

New training method helps surgeons evaluate their own minimally invasive surgery skills

Recent years have seen the rapid emergence of minimally invasive surgery procedures in operating theatres. However, the training of surgeons in this field still leaves much to be desired.

Researcher Magdalena Chmarra has changed this state of affairs by developing a realistic training system which records and analyses the surgeon's movements. As a result there is now, for the first time, an objective benchmark for measuring a surgeon's basic skills in the field of minimally invasive surgery. Chmarra will receive her PhD for this research at Delft University of Technology in The Netherlands on Monday 12 January.

Despite its considerable advantages, the relatively recent technique of minimally invasive surgery still has a number of drawbacks. One such disadvantage relates to the training of surgeons, which is still, for the most part, delivered in a rather unstructured manner and, moreover, without any objective benchmark with which to measure the progress made by trainee surgeons.

Training

Broadly speaking, there are currently two safe training methods for minimally invasive surgery. The first is the so-called box trainer, an enclosed rectangular box in which trainee surgeons can practise performing basic manipulative tasks with the surgical devices, such as picking up and moving objects. As they do this, they can be assessed by an experienced surgeon. Clearly, this is a somewhat subjective process.

The other option is the virtual reality trainer, employing computer simulations, which allows for excellent recording and analysis of the surgeon's actions. However, this training method still has the major disadvantage that it lacks realism. For example, users feel no tactile response when performing surgical tasks.

TrEndo

Thus both of these training methods have their drawbacks. The Delft doctoral candidate Magdalena Chmarra has sought to change this situation by developing a training tool that is realistic for the surgeon and at the same time records and analyses the motion of the instruments manipulated by the surgeon. This is accomplished with an inexpensive and relatively simple tracking device known as the 'TrEndo'. A TrEndo incorporates three optical computer-mouse sensors which record the movements made by the surgeon in all directions.

9 Powering pacemakers

Read the text. Work in pairs to answer the questions.

1 Which two of these are mentioned as findings of the Southampton study?
   a Harvesting surplus energy caused considerable damage to the heart in some people.
   b As the heart increased so did the energy harvested for the microgenerator.
   c The amount of energy harvested was very erratic.
   d Increases in the energy harvested still rose when the blood pressure was reduced.
   e The lining of the heart's chambers was not noticeably damaged by implanting the microgenerator.

2 Which of these two predictions about the findings of the Southampton study does Roberts make?
   a Pacemakers might soon have much smaller working parts.
   b The capability of pacemakers could be increased.
   c Pacemakers could be powered indefinitely by micrognerators.
   d Pacemakers will save the lives of everyone fitted with the devices.

3 Which two of these are mentioned as drawbacks of the increase in battery size to power the devices?
   a The discomfort
   b The cost
   c The shape
   d The weight
   e The thickness

4 What is the current focus of the researchers?

Heart's surplus energy may help power pacemakers, defibrillators

In an experimental study researchers show a beating heart may produce enough energy to power a pacemaker or defibrillator.

NEW ORLEANS, LA., Nov. 10, 2008 – Surplus energy generated by the heart may one day help power pacemakers and defibrillators implanted in cardiac patients, according to research presented at the American Heart Association's Scientific Sessions 2008.

In a trailblazing experiment, a microgenerator powered by heartbeats produced almost 17 per cent of the electricity needed to run an artificial pacemaker. 'This was a proof-of-concept study, and we proved the concept,' said Paul Roberts, MD, first author of the study and a Consultant Electrophysiologist at Southampton University Hospital in the United Kingdom. 'Harvesting surplus energy might be a major transition in implantable pacemakers and defibrillators because engineers will have more energy to work with.'

In their study, researchers found:

- At a heart rate of 80 beats per minute (bpm), the device yielded an average harvested energy of 4.3 microjoules per cardiac cycle.
- Increasing changes in the heart rate produced corresponding increases in energy. At 104 to 128 bpm, the harvested energy level increased 140 per cent.
- Decreases occurred when the researchers slowed the heartbeat or lowered blood pressure.
- Implantation and surplus energy harvesting caused no significant injury to the lining of the heart's chambers.

'What this might mean is that in the next era of pacemakers, you'd get devices that lasted significantly longer and we could add more functions to help monitor the heart,' Roberts said. 'It's possible they could be efficient enough to allow complete and indefinite powering of pacemakers.' Since their introduction into clinical medicine, implantable pacemakers and defibrillators have saved lives and become more sophisticated. However, adding new monitoring capabilities to the devices has led designers to a critical point.

'The small devices now are really very good, but power consumption must increase if we want to take them to the next level,' Roberts said. 'Battery technology has plateaued and the only way we are going to increase power is to increase size.' This, in turn, would increase the units' weight, making them more uncomfortable and less cosmetically acceptable to patients because the devices are implanted under the skin.

The innovative generator – called the self-energizing implantable medical microsystem (SIMM) – helps the heart produce more than enough energy with each beat to pump blood. The SIMM uses two compressible bladders and a microgenerator mounted on the lead of a pacemaker or defibrillator, the wire that connects the device to the heart. The lead is attached to the end of the right ventricle, and the bladders relay the energy from the pressure of each heartbeat to the microgenerator, which transforms it into electricity for use by the battery.

A consortium of companies including InVivo Technology, Perpetuum and Zarlink Semiconductor developed and tested the SIMM microgenerator with United Kingdom government funds. Researchers used an in-vivo porcine model to evaluate the study. The researchers are now working to improve the materials used in the SIMM microgenerator.

'With different materials, we're seeing even greater energy harvesting,' Roberts said. 'While at the moment we see about twenty per cent harvesting, we're anticipating that will be significantly more in the next iteration of the device.'

10 Ethical issues

1 Work in pairs. What ethical issues do you think might arise in the field of respiratory medicine? Give examples from your own experience.

2 Read the text. Work in groups and as quickly as you can find nouns that are connected in meaning with these verbs.

1 make worse
2 suit
3 lengthen
4 revive
5 necessitate
6 limit
7 differ

3 Answer the questions.

1 What arise at the end of a patient's life?
2 What can the effect of artificial ventilation sometimes be?
3 What can the patient ask for even if the medical team denies treatment?
4 When should decisions about resuscitation and formal ventilation be taken?
5 What does not improve respiratory acidosis?

Ethical issues

Most ethical issues faced by doctors arise at the end of a patient's life. This particularly applies to respiratory physicians, where difficult decisions about the appropriateness of treatment and the prolongation of life in patients with chronic underlying lung diseases may need to be made. In some situations artificial ventilation may prolong the dying process; life has a natural end and the potential to prolong life in the intensive care unit can sometimes cause dilemmas.

The General Medical Council (GMC) in the UK states that doctors have an obligation to respect human life, protect the health of their patients, and put their patients' best interests first. This means offering treatment where the benefits outweigh any risks, and avoiding treatments that carry no net gain to the patient. If a patient wishes to have a treatment that in the doctor's considered view is not indicated, the doctor and medical team are under no ethical or legal obligation to provide it (but the patient's right to a second opinion must be respected).

The decision about resuscitation and formal ventilation is never an easy one, but should ideally be taken with the nursing staff, the patient, and their next of kin, in advance of an emergency situation. In practical terms, this is clearly not always possible. Ideally, all decisions regarding resuscitation and the ceiling of treatment (particularly relating to ventilation) should be documented in advance and handed over to the on-call team. Most possible outcomes can be anticipated.

Where it is decided the treatment is not in the best interests of

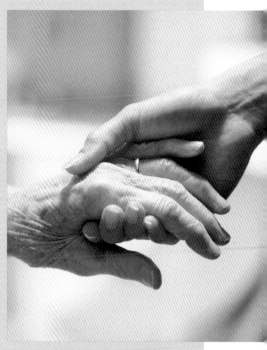

the patient, there is no ethical distinction between stopping the treatment or not starting it in the first place (though the former may be more difficult to do), and this should be used as an argument for failing to initiate the treatment in the first place.

Some clinical scenarios are more commonly encountered by the respiratory physician. COPD is the fourth commonest cause of death in America and most patients die of respiratory failure during an exacerbation. A commonly encountered clinical situation is where a patient with COPD is admitted with an exacerbation, and it is type II respiratory failure. Standard treatment does not improve respiratory acidosis, so non-invasive ventilation is commenced. Before starting NIV, a decision must be clearly documented as to whether or not NIV is the ceiling treatment. It may be if the patient has severe or end stage COPD.

11 Coping in the tropics

1 Work in groups. Have you ever worked in difficult conditions where you had to 'sleep rough'? Give examples. If you haven't, how do you think you would cope?

2 Read the text. In groups, complete the text using a–g.

a you risk cuts, insect bites or snake bites, larva migrans, jiggers, etc.

b to preserve comfort and skin

c at night they become much cooler, and travellers in upland forests may require a blanket or lightweight sleeping bag

d there is a potential source of infections such as histoplasmosis and Chagas' disease

e this is best cleared from the ground beneath hammocks and around tent entrances

f they protect against sawgrass cuts, especially when using a machete

g ensure that boots are properly worn in before entering the jungle

Tropical forests

Tropical rainforests cover a dwindling six per cent of the earth's land mass and are defined by their location (between the Tropic of Cancer 23° 27' N and the Tropic of Capricorn 23° 27' S) and their high rainfall, which can be several metres a year. During the day, the forests are hot and humid, often with little breeze to give respite, but ¹_____. The forest floor may be underwater for much of the year. Primary rainforest, where the high tree canopy suppresses ground growth, is more open than secondary forest. Here previous felling allows light to reach the forest floor and promote growth of dense jungle.

Clothing and footwear

- Accept daytime wetness. Rinse kit in camp and re-wear wet next day. Keep a dry set of clothing in a plastic bag for evening and bedtime use ²_____.
- Never go barefoot or wear sandals as ³_____.
- Use boots with good treads that dry quickly. De-roofed blisters could develop into ulcers, so ⁴_____.
- Cover up as long sleeves and trousers protect you from irritant plants and insect bites.
- Wear gloves as ⁵_____.
- Wear a hat to protect you against the sun, rain, and barbed leaves.

Bases and campsites

Choose with care:

- Avoid river banks, which can flash flood from distant rains upstream. Low river banks are access points to and from the water for wild animals. Check potential campsite for animal spoor and droppings.
- Avoid abandoned local shelters. They may be structurally unsound and can harbour spiders, ants, rodents, and snakes which feed off them. Even when the fauna has left, ⁶_____.
- Look up: site shelters away from rotting trees or branches that could crash down (so-called 'deadfall').
- Sleep off the ground to avoid snakes, scorpions, etc. Construct a raised sleeping platform or sling hammock. Use a mosquito net and, if outside, protect yourself from rain using plastic sheeting or tarpaulin.

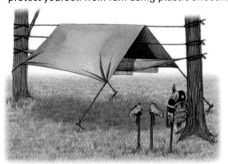

- Clearing enough ground for tents can take a lot of energy and it can be difficult to remove stumps effectively. If used, tents should have a midge mesh, sewn in bucket type ground sheet and zips that seal the entrance. They can be stiflingly hot and are heavy when wet.
- Leaf litter can hide snakes and scorpions, so ⁷_____.
- Protect group areas from rain by tarpaulin.

12 Smart fabrics

1 Work in pairs. Which of the following do you think are the most likely uses of technology in 'smart (medical) clothing'?

- temperature control
- monitoring a baby and the mother during pregnancy
- monitoring the heart
- detecting illness
- collecting general medical data

2 Read the text. In pairs, complete the text using a–h.

a crucial hurdles
b a recuperative break
c challenging problems
d a serious work safety issue
e a smart fabric
f typical electronics
g muscle fatigue
h a mature field of research

3 Work in pairs. Underline the correct alternative to make the sentences true.

1 According to the writer, smart fabric research is *in its infancy / old technology / not worth investing in*.

2 The use of clever clothing is being held back by its *lack of dependability and obtrusiveness / dependability alone / obtrusiveness alone*.

3 Among the potential users of smart fabrics in clothing are *dancers / singers / sportspeople*.

4 RSI is mainly caused by small amounts of stress over a *short / long / modest* period of time

5 Measuring the heart is affected by the *sound / electricity / heat* produced by the clothes moving.

4 Work in groups. What would you like to see smart clothing used for in the medical field? Give reasons and examples.

Smart fabrics make clever (medical) clothing

EUROPEAN researchers have developed [1]_____ that can monitor muscular overload and help prevent repetitive strain injury, or RSI. But that is just the beginning. The team is also exploring a pregnancy belt to monitor a baby's heartbeat, clothing to help coach hockey, and shirts that monitor [2]_____ during training.

Smart fabrics promise to revolutionize clothing by incorporating sensors into cloth for health, lifestyle, and business applications. In the long term, they could consist of circuits and sensors that provide all of the [3]_____ we carry around today, like mobile phones and PDAs.

Current, first-generation applications are far more modest, and pioneering medical smart fabrics are used to monitor vital signs like heart rate and temperature. But two [4]_____ – unobtrusiveness and reliability – impede widespread adoption of such clever clothes.

Now one European research team has developed groundbreaking medical-sensing smart fabrics, and its work could lead to pregnancy monitoring belts, sports clothing that provides training tips, a wearable physical game controller, and a vest that helps to prevent repetitive strain injury.

The Context project initially sought to develop an RSI vest to tackle [5]_____. Repetitive actions can, over time, lead to permanent injury and the problem costs billions of euros a year. It affects over 40 million workers across the continent and is responsible for 50 per cent of all work-related ill-health.

Muscle contraction, the very quiet metric

The team had to tackle three [6]_____. First, they were using a relatively novel sensor that demanded sophisticated electronics located in the clothing. Second, they were aiming to measure muscle contraction, a very 'quiet metric'. Third, they were venturing on a research path seldom trodden: muscle contraction as a predictor for stress. Long-term, low-key stress is the leading risk factor for RSI.

'Each of the issues was very difficult. We chose to use a capacitative sensor, because it does not need to be attached to the skin like resistive sensors do, which adds to the comfort. It needs controlling electronics close to the sensor to work effectively, and that presents a real challenge for textile integration,' explains Bas Feddes, Context's co-ordinator.

Similarly, measuring electromyography, or electrical activity in the muscle, is more subtle and tricky than electrocardiography, which measures the heart. The rustle of clothing caused by movement can drown out the signal. Context has gone a long way to solving that problem but it is not as robust as they would like.

Finally, medical understanding of muscle stress as a predictor for RSI is not [7]_____, so it is difficult to say with certainty that specific activities could lead to RSI. Despite these hurdles, the team successfully designed an RSI vest, and they are currently improving its reliability.

Context's ambitious programme tackled pioneering and very complex issues in smart-fabric research, which resulted in a useful, unobtrusive, and reliable RSI vest that can warn wearers to take [8]_____.

Reading bank key

1 Triage

1 Students' own answers.

2 1 life-threatening
2 categories
3 red
4 non-urgent / blue

3 1 a senior, experienced individual with considerable common sense. Note that *dedicated* means 'assigned only to that duty'.
2 elevating injured limbs, applying ice packs or splints, and giving analgesia
3 no more than a few minutes
4 because the urgency (and hence the triage category) with which a patient requires to be seen may change with time
5 standard to very urgent

4 non-urgent categories, inordinately long periods, perceived to be more urgent, aware of this, Uncomplaining elderly patients.

2 Preventing injuries

1 Students' own answers.

2 1 load
2 prevent
3 identify
4 struck
5 recommends
6 detach
7 attached
8 dismounted
9 inspect
10 pronounced

3 1 relates to hydraulic excavators and backhoe loaders
2 suggests two common causes of injury
3 Other leading causes of fatalities are …
4 He was pronounced dead at the scene
5 … toward the victim standing in the trench

3 How dangerous is skiing?

1 1c 2e 3a 4d 5b

2 1 game of football
2 spatial awareness
3 topography
4 risks
5 collisions

3 Students' own answers.

4 Fathers and pregnancy

1 Students' own answers.

2 1d 2f 3c 4e 5g 6b 7a

3 Students' own answers.

5 OCD

1 Students' own answers.

2 1 Yes
2 No
3 Yes
4 Yes
5 No
6 No
7 No

3 2 It affects 2–3% of the population.
5 as well as those of healthy close relatives (a sibling, parent, or child)
6 Participants also completed a computerized test.
7 Both OCD patients and their close relatives fared worse on the computer task than the control group.

4 1 unrelated
2 household
3 prevalent
4 distinctive
5 repetitive
6 similar
7 improved
8 contributing
9 underlying

6 Nifty after fifty

1 Students' own answers.

2 1 deteriorating
2 popping up
3 work out
4 frenetic
5 intimidated
6 homing in on
7 limber
8 mushroomed
9 disposable
10 pulls in

3 1 John Atwood
2 International Health, Racquet & Sportsclub Association
3 Sheldon Zinberg
4 National Association of Area Agencies on Ageing
5 John Atwood

4 Students' own answers.

7 Roman face cream

1 Students' own answers.

2 1 discovered
2 complete
3 stunned to discover what was inside
4 do not normally survive
5 Tests to be carried out soon
6 said that the offering may well have been made
7 be converted to homes, offices, and shops

3 1 What was uncovered lately?
2 What condition were the contents of the tin in?
3 What was the reaction of the experts when they opened the tin?
4 What normally happens to Roman cream?
5 What will be performed in the near future?
6 Who did historians propose made the donation?
7 What will happen to the archaeological site?

4 Students' own answers.

8 Training for surgeons

1 Students' own answers.

2 1 feel no tactile response
2 an objective benchmark
3 a somewhat subjective process
4 it lacks realism
5 has changed this state of affairs
6 still has a number of drawbacks
7 leaves much to be desired

3 1 the (rapid) emergence of minimally invasive surgery procedures in operating theatres
2 the unstructured training of surgeons and lack of any objective benchmark to measure trainee progress
3 two: the so-called box trainer and the virtual reality trainer
4 subjective, lack of realism, and no tactile response
5 It records and analyses the motion of the instruments manipulated by the surgeon

4 Students' own answers.

9 Powering pacemakers

1 b and e

2 b and c

3 a and d

4 to improve the materials used in the SIMM microgenerator

10 Ethical issues

1 Students' own answers.

2 1 exacerbation
2 appropriateness
3 prolongation
4 resuscitation
5 obligation
6 ceiling
7 distinction

3 1 most ethical issues
2 prolong the dying process
3 a second opinion
4 in advance of an emergency situation
5 standard treatment

11 Coping in the tropics

1 Students' own answers.

2 1c 2b 3a 4g 5f 6d 7e

12 Smart fabrics

1 Students' own answers.

2 1e 2g 3f 4a 5d 6c 7h 8b

3 1 in its infancy
2 lack of dependability and obtrusiveness
3 sportspeople
4 long
5 sound

4 Students' own answers.

7 Dermatology

Check up

1 Work in groups. Describe the pictures and identify the types of skin condition shown.

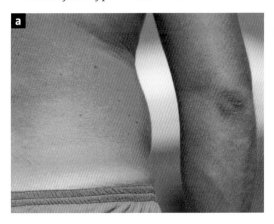

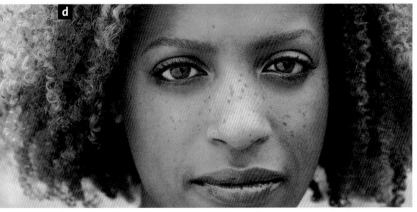

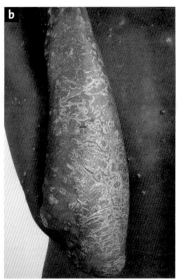

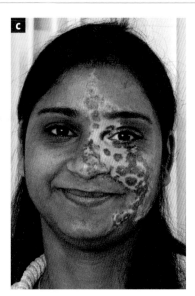

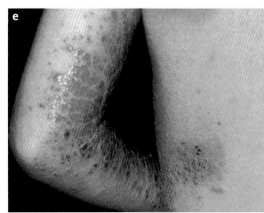

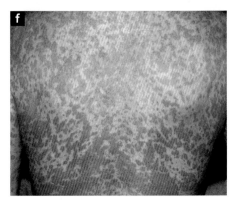

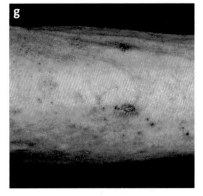

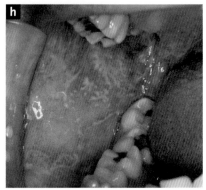

2 What are the causes of each?

3 Why are dermatological problems especially distressing?

4 What experience have you had of treating dermatological conditions?

Vocabulary

Lesions

1 Work in pairs. What lesions do the diagrams show? When you have answered as many as you can, look at the list at the bottom to help you.

a
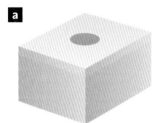
Flat, non-palpable change in skin-colour <0.5cm

b
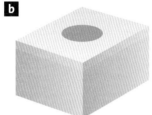
Flat, non-palpable change in skin-colour >0.5cm

c
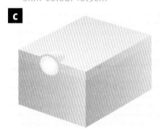
Fluid below the epidermis

d
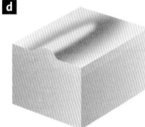
Dermal oedema

e
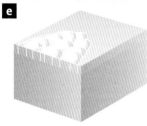
A small thin piece of horny epithelium resembling that of a fish

f
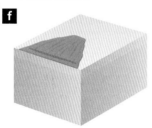
Dried exudate is a crust of blood / plasma

g
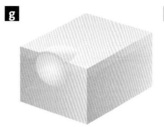
Visible collection of pus in the subcutis

h
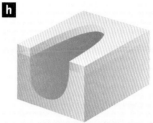
Full thickness skin loss

i
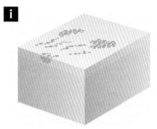
A rash caused by blood in the skin – often multiple petechiae

j
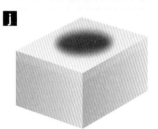
A 'bruise'. Technically a form of purpura

crust	ecchimosis	macule	patch
purpura	pustule	ulcer	vesicle
wheal	scale		

2 In groups, discuss how you distinguish between lesions, for example, between a wheal and a plaque? Give an example of a condition in which you would see each of these lesions.

3 Which lesions would you associate with these verbs: *itch, ooze, discharge, spread, scab, harden*?

Listening 1

Listening for details

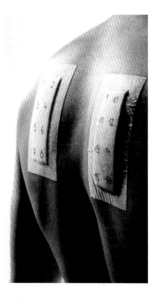

1 🎧 Listen to the extract of a conversation between Dr Jackson and John Dodds. Write as many details as possible. You may have to listen twice.

2 Work in pairs. One student reads their notes to their partner and they check any differences.

3 🎧 Listen again and check for detail.

4 Can you improve on the doctor's questions?

5 Map the doctor's questions: open, closed, leading, etc.

6 What other reassuring statements could the doctor have used?

7 Which diagram in *Vocabulary* matches the conversation?

Patient care

1 Work in pairs. Match the two parts of the patients' statements.

1 I found the whole experience so distressing

2 I couldn't leave it alone. I just kept playing with it

3 It scabbed over and I picked at it and made it bleed. I know

4 I know it's covered up

5 I keep telling him to leave it alone

6 I suppose a lot of people would be bothered by it,

7 I'm almost beside myself with it;

8 My husband says it's only a few white patches,

9 I've come out in these little red spots

a but I don't really care.

b but I'm worried about them.

c and there are a lot more unsightly things than this, but I am always aware of it.

d I shouldn't have but I couldn't help it.

e here on both my wrists and elbows. They're really itchy and irritating.

f I don't know if I have ever been so distressed in my life.

g I'm just worried that it will leave scars on my face.

h and I couldn't stop myself from scratching.

i and stop rubbing it, but he's just very worked up by it.

2 Find words and expressions in **1** that mean the same as these.

1 form a crust
2 play about with
3 ugly
4 conscious
5 agitated
6 terrified
7 blemish
8 macule
9 cicatrix

3 In which sentences in **1** is the patient very upset?

4 When the patient says something that indicates how they feel, it is important to be able to acknowledge the cues given by the patient. These cues may be verbal, visual, intuitive, or aural. You need to acknowledge them to show that you are listening and then follow them up with reassurance. Choose two or more statements in **1** and decide how you would reassure the patient.

USEFUL EXPRESSIONS

It sounds / looks / seems as if ...
You sound / look / seem ... (if I am right?)
The treatment can make it look worse than it is.
With children, it's difficult to stop them scratching.
You must have (been itching a lot with this).

5 Work in pairs. Take turns reassuring each other.

6 Still in pairs use one or more of the other statements in **1** to do a role-play without any preparation.

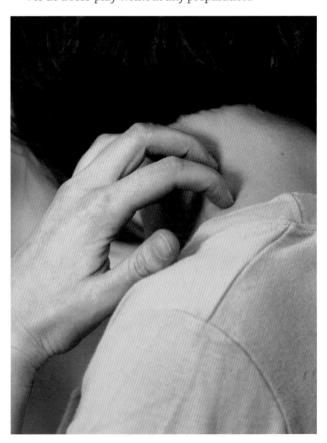

rash (n) eruption of the skin in spots or patches
flare up (v) erupt

● **Language spot**
Commenting on the past

1 Work in pairs. Correct the sentences where necessary.

1 I must've knocked my arm on something and then these lumps have come up.
2 I should've come sooner and then the rash would be so bad.
3 I should've put anything on as that's what's made it flare up.
4 When I was stung, I could go into shock. I wish I'd known.
5 He didn't need to pay for his treatment.
6 Surely, I can't have pick up scabies.
7 I would come earlier, but I had to take the children to school.
8 I should've pay closer attention and kept the box the tablets were in.
9 Yes, you're right. It should've cleared up by now.
10 Shouldn't it have go by now?
11 I needn't have paid for the prescription.

2 Which of the statements in **1** describe things that did not take place?

3 What would be the effect on the patient if the doctor said: *You should've paid attention to what you were doing and ...; you shouldn't have used that cream...*

4 Think of three things that you have done recently or you haven't done recently. Describe them to a partner.

USEFUL EXPRESSIONS
What I should(n't) have done was ...
What I could have done was ...
I needn't have / I didn't need to ..., but ...
I would've ... but I couldn't ...

≫ Go to **Grammar reference** p 123

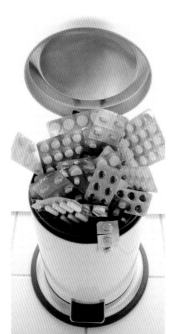

Speaking

1 Identify the two skin conditions and give reasons for your diagnosis.

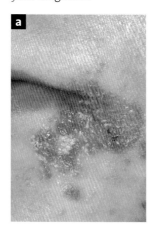
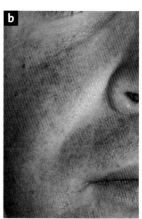

a impetigo
b acne rosacea

2 Work in groups. Prepare a role-play. A patient is going to present with a skin complaint. Make a list of the questions you would ask the patient under these headings:

The presenting complaint
Past medical history
Allergies
Drug history
Family history
Social history
Psychosocial impact

3 Compare your list with another group or the rest of the class.

4 Work in pairs. Student A, go to page 114. Student B, go to page 116. In the role-play, the patient answers the doctor's questions according to the diagnosis of the skin condition on the picture. The patient shows the picture to the 'doctor' at the appropriate moment. Make sure the doctor does not see the picture with the diagnosis.

5 When you finish, check how many questions in exercise **2** you asked.

6 Give feedback on your own and your partner's performance.

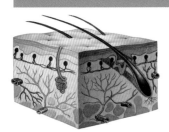

Cross-section of the skin

Reading

1 Before you read the text, work in pairs. Answer these questions.

1 What functions does the skin perform?
2 What are the layers of the skin?
3 What functions do glands perform?

2 Find words in the text which are made from these:

1 society   3 sight   5 lie   7 mix
2 thesis   4 out   6 append   8 number

3 Look at these answers. Read the text and decide what questions you would ask for each one.

1 the integumentary system
2 prevention of water loss, antigen presentation, and sensation
3 unsightly blemishes
4 about three months
5 the superficial fascia
6 puberty

Applied anatomy and physiology

The skin, nails, hair, glands, and associated nerve endings make up the 'integumentary system'.

Skin

The skin acts as a physical, biochemical, and immunological barrier between the outside world and the body. It also has a role in temperature regulation, synthesis of vitamin D, prevention of water loss, antigen presentation, and sensation.

It is important to remember that the skin also has an important psychosocial function. When we look at another person, we are in fact looking at their skin. As our skin represents our outward appearance to the world, unsightly blemishes, despite their small size, can have a significant impact on a person's self esteem.

The skin is made up of three layers – epidermis, dermis, and hypodermis.

Epidermis

This is the outermost layer and is formed of a modified stratified squamous epithelium.

Almost 90% of epithelial cells are keratinocytes. These cells are produced in the basal layer and then rise to the surface as more are produced below and the outer cells are shed. The time taken from forming in the basal layer to shedding is usually about three months.

Melanocytes reside in the basal layer and secrete melanin into surrounding keratinocytes via long projections. This, along with the underlying fat and blood, gives the skin its colour. In this way, skin tone is determined by the size and number of melanin granules and not by the number of melanocytes.

Dermis

Below the epidermis lies a layer of connective tissue consisting of collagen, elastic fibres, and ground substance. It is here where the 'skin appendages', muscles, nerves, and blood vessels lie.

Hypodermis

Also known as the subcutaneous layer or the superficial fascia, this consists of adipose tissue and serves both as a lipid store and provides insulation. It also contributes to the body contours and shape.

Glands

After infancy, sebaceous glands become active again at puberty and secrete sebum, a mixture of fatty acids and salts, directly onto the skin or into the necks of hair follicles. This waterproofs and lubricates the skin and hair. They are particularly numerous in the upper chest, back, face, and scalp.

Sweat glands secrete a mixture of water, electrolytes, urea, urate, ammonia, and mild acids. Eccrine sweat glands are found all over the body surface, besides the mucosa. Apocrine sweat glands are found in the axillae and pubic regions, secrete a more viscous sweat, and are under clear autonomic control. These do not function until puberty.

4 Work in groups. Describe a case where you dealt with a patient with a dermatological complaint and where you feel that you could've / should've / couldn't have done things differently.

angry (adj) red / inflamed

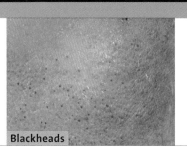

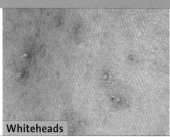

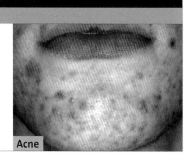

Blackheads

Whiteheads

Acne

Listening 2
Dealing with teenagers

1 Work in groups. Look at this scenario. What would have been the management and what advice do you think should have been given? Make a list.

> A sixteen-year-old male patient, Brian Collins, presented with spots on his face, neck, back, and chest. Examination reveals blackheads (comedones) and whiteheads, red papules, pustules, and cysts.

2 🎧 Listen to an extract from the consultation after the doctor, Dr Aimee Preston, has examined the patient. Check which items on your list were mentioned and add those which were not.

3 🎧 Listen again. Answer the questions and say how the doctor does it in each case.
1 Is the doctor sympathetic?
2 Is the doctor reassuring?
3 Is the language simple?
4 Does the doctor seek cooperation?
5 Does the doctor seek to ensure compliance?
6 Does the doctor warn the patient about the duration of the treatment?
7 Does the doctor seek to involve the patient in the management?
8 Does the doctor use 'safety netting'?
9 Does the doctor arrange a follow-up?

4 🎧 Compare notes with partner and if necessary listen again.

5 Work in pairs. Take turns talking to the patient in the scenario in 1 above.

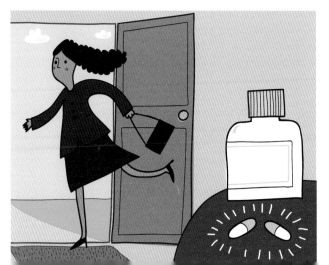

● Language spot
Verbs with *to* and *-ing*

1 Look at this extract from *Listening 2* and underline the verbs in the *-ing* form. Can you use the infinitive with *to* instead?

> *... and I don't like going out as people look at it and I think it's dirty. And it keeps getting worse. I've tried cutting out certain foods, but nothing works, and using different creams and stuff.*

2 Complete the sentences using the *-ing* form or the *to*-infinitive of the verbs in brackets. There may be more than one possible answer for some items.
1 I have to admit to _____ (not use) the ointment you gave me.
2 I stopped _____ (apply) the cream because it made my skin very angry looking.
3 I forgot _____ (make) an appointment to see the nurse.
4 Yes. I remember _____ (get) the medicine.
5 I always avoid _____ (sit) in the sun.
6 I regret not _____ (come) in sooner.
7 I didn't finish _____ (take) the medication.
8 I meant _____ (apply) it every morning, but it meant _____ (get up) earlier and it made me late for work.
9 Following the treatment requires _____ (plan) and a lot of effort.

3 Work in pairs. Take turns being the doctor and a patient with acne. The patient should choose at least three of the statements above. The doctor should give a response and develop the conversation.

USEFUL EXPRESSIONS
Yes. It's not easy ...   It takes time ...
Do you think you could ... ?   Is there any way round this ... ?
Was there any particular reason ... ?

≫ Go to **Grammar reference** p 123

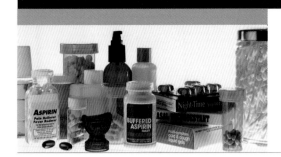

Pronunciation

Main stress in a sentence

1 🎧 Listen to the patient speaking. Write the exact words that the patient says.

2 Compare your answers with a partner.

3 🎧 Listen again and mark the main stress in the sentence. If you need to, listen for a third time.

4 Practise saying the statements to each other. Did your partner say all the syllables?

5 Follow the same procedure as in *Language spot* 3. This time concentrate on the pronunciation.

It's my job

1 Before you read, discuss this question in pairs.
- What do you think is the value of the practice nurse in helping patients stick to their treatment?

2 Read the text and answer the questions.
1 How did Zahra become interested in dermatology?
2 Why do you think skin problems might be particularly upsetting for children and teenagers?
3 What two things can help patients with skin problems?
4 What is the difference between compliance and concordance?
5 How does Zahra encourage a patient to follow a regime?

3 Work in groups. Describe cases where you know that you have been successful in encouraging patients to keep to a treatment regime. Say why you were successful.

4 What are the main factors affecting compliance in your country or where you are working?

Zahra El-Ashry

My name is Zahra El-Ashry. I'm a practice nurse working in a GP surgery, and I've got a postgraduate diploma in dermatology. I became interested in this particular area when I saw how distressed people were when they came to the surgery where I work with various skin problems. It's bad enough for adults, but for children and teenagers it's particularly upsetting.

Sometimes, just a few words help to make things better. But the main thing is help with the treatment itself as it is sometimes complex. It is easy to get annoyed at the patient's poor compliance until you reframe this as a lack of concordance; then we as health professionals may get annoyed with ourselves which is just as bad. In order to encourage the patient to comply with any regimen that the doctor agrees with the patient, we have found that concordance works if the patient sees me after the doctor to help in planning treatment through dialogue and understanding lifestyle constraints. We have found from talking to other practices that nurses are invaluable in demonstrating topical therapies and in optimizing concordance.

Project

Work in groups. Each group chooses one of the items below. Check the suggested sources and use your own experience to collect information on the management of the condition. You may check information with students in other groups. Look at these websites:

1 psoriasis: www.psoriasis-association-org.uk
2 eczema: www. eczema.org.uk
3 solar keratosis: www.SkinCancer.org
4 Also check www.patient.co.uk
5 Electronic Dermatology Atlas www.Dermis.net for photosensitivity / sunlight and the skin

Speaking

1 Work in groups. Collate the information from *Project* that you collected about your chosen topic. Create a scenario with which you are going to test fellow students in another group. In the scenarios you may choose to take a history and discuss the management, or discuss only the management with a patient. Give the patient: *a name, an age, an attitude, a level of anxiety.* Discuss how the patient will think and react to the diagnosis and management. Write down the scenario on a piece of paper.

2 As a group, go though the information for the scenario once quickly.

3 Work with a partner from another group with a different scenario. Choose who should go first. Give your partner the paper with your scenario on it. Take turns taking the history and discussing the management or discussing the management only. Use the checklist on page 117 and choose at least two criteria for your partner to use to assess your performance, e.g. *reassurance, sympathy, empathy, being patient centred.*

Remember to be reassuring, sympathetic, and empathetic.

USEFUL EXPRESSIONS
You must have been ...
We need to be patient ...
It takes time to work ...
It looks / seems / sounds ...

Writing

Reflection on professional experience

1 Work in groups. Talk about the decisions you have made in your career so far. In your consideration, talk about whether you should have chosen or would choose dermatology as a specialty.

2 Within your group, describe cases where you treated a patient with a dermatological problem. Explain what happened and say how you would improve on what you did. Give examples of what you should have and shouldn't have done and say what you learnt from it. Remember to maintain patient confidentiality.

3 When you apply for jobs, you may be asked to give examples of your own experience and what you have learnt from it. Using your own ideas only, write between 150 and 200 words describing the case in **2** and remember to say what you learnt from it.

Checklist

Assess your progress in this unit.
Tick (✓) the statements which are true.

I can comment on the past

I can use verbs with *to* or *-ing*

I can talk about dermatology

I can understand patient language

I can understand patients at natural speed

Key words

Adjective
psychosocial

Nouns
acne (vulgaris)
blemish
compliance
concordance
crust
cue
dermatology
purpura
scab
vesicle
wheal

Verbs
avoid
itch
keep
mean
pick at
play with
stop

Useful reference

Oxford Handbook of Clinical Examination and Practical Skills, Thomas and Monaghan (eds), ISBN 978-019-856838-4

8 Surgery

Check up

1 Work in groups. Describe the pictures.

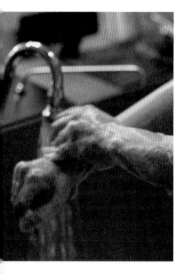
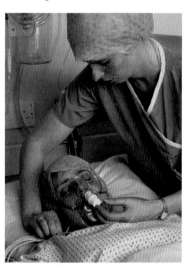
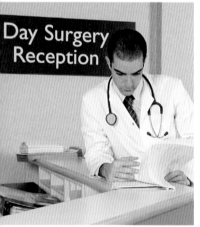
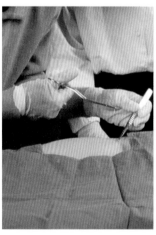

2 What is involved in scrubbing up prior to an operation? How do you gown and glove?

3 Have you ever practised doing sutures on manikins? What manikins have you used?

4 What minor / major operations have you performed or been present at?

5 What are the benefits of day-case surgery to the patient, the surgeon, and the hospital? Is day-case surgery common in your country?

Vocabulary
Medical terminology for surgery

1 Match the prefixes with their meanings.

1	laparo-	a	nose
2	nephro-	b	breast
3	pyelo-	c	large bowel
4	cysto-	d	chest
5	chole-	e	uterus
6	col(on)-	f	bile / the biliary system
7	hystero-	g	kidney
8	thoraco-	h	abdomen
9	rhino-	i	renal pelvis
10	masto- / mammo-	j	bladder

2 Complete the sentences by combining one of the prefixes above with one of the suffixes below. You may use some of the suffixes more than once.

-ectomy   -lithotomy   -pexy   -plasty
-r(h)aphy,   -ostomy   -otomy

1 We're going to do something called a _____ to have a look inside your tummy.

2 I'm afraid we're going to have to do an operation called a _____ to remove your right kidney.

3 The only option left to us is a _____, where we remove part of your large bowel and then make an opening in your tummy wall.

4 So how do you feel about having your womb removed by laparoscopic _____?

5 We're going to do a procedure which will involve a _____, where we remove several ribs.

6 We can do bilateral _____, where we lift both breasts.

7 We can do a _____, where we stitch the bladder.

8 We're going to have to remove the gall bladder. The technical name for this operation is _____.

9 What we're going to do is destroy some stones in the kidney in a procedure called _____.

10 We're going to do a procedure called a _____ to fix the large part of your gut.

Pronunciation

Secondary stress

Words that are polysyllabic usually have a nucleus and a secondary stress.

1 Look at the words in *Vocabulary* **2**, and in pairs decide where the nucleus and secondary stress occur.

2 🎧 Listen. Circle the nucleus and underline the secondary stress of each word where appropriate.

1 ●●○●●	6 ●●●●	
2 ●●●●	7 ●●●●	
3 ●●●●	8 ●●●●●●●	
4 ●●●●●	9 ●●●●●●●●	
5 ●●●●●	10 ●●●●	

3 Work in pairs. Using the sentences in *Vocabulary* **2**, take turns informing each other what operation is going to be done.

Listening 1

Patient response

1 🎧 Listen to the conversation between Dr Irina Petrov and Mr Blackstone. Decide whether the patient is apprehensive or relaxed about the operation.

2 🎧 Listen again. Answer the questions below and note down evidence.

1 Which adjectives describe the doctor's manner / tone during the conversation?

brusque	*caring*	*friendly*
honest	*patronizing*	*reassuring*

2 Is the doctor patient centred? Does she involve the patient in the decision making?
3 Does the doctor give the patient a chance to ask questions?
4 Is the information presented in a way that the patient can understand? How?
5 Does the doctor ask about consent for the operation?
6 Does the doctor explain the operation clearly?
7 Does the doctor check that the patient understands?
8 Is the doctor reassuring about the pain?
9 Is the doctor aware throughout of the patient's feelings?

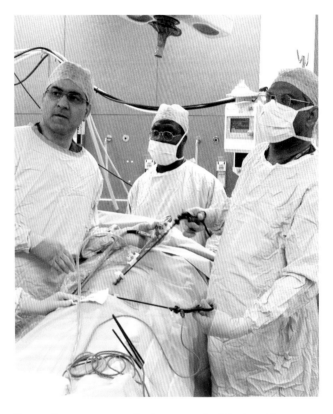

3 Work in groups. Study this scenario. What are the similarities between this scenario and the scenario in **1** from the communication point of view? What is the father likely to feel?

A 35-year-old father presents with a seven-year-old child, Arthur, who has perforated appendix. Explain to the father that the child has to have an emergency operation. Explain what you think it is and explain that an operation is necessary.

USEFUL EXPRESSIONS
Arthur's got what is ...
We can do an operation called a ..., where we ...
What we do is ...
How do you feel about Arthur having the operation?
We'll need you to sign a consent form if you're happy with everything.
Is there anything you'd like to ask me?

4 Choose two people in your group to role-play the scenario while the others watch. Use the questions in **2** as a checklist to give feedback.

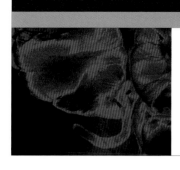

X-ray of appendix
and colon

• **Language spot**

Relative pronouns in explanations

Work in pairs. Connect the sentences using one or more
of the words in brackets and / or 'zero relative'. You will
need to add and remove some words.

EXAMPLE
*Herniorrhaphy's an operation. It's done under local or
general anaesthetic. The muscle in the tummy wall is
strengthened using a special mesh. (where / when)*

*Herniorrhaphy's an operation, done under local or
general anaesthetic, where the muscle in the tummy
wall is strengthened using a special mesh.*

1 We're going to do something. It is called a
 mastectomy. A breast is removed. (when / where)

2 It's a type of stitch. It is done under the skin so that
 there is only a faint scar left at the end. The wound
 heals. (which / when)

3 A colostomy is a procedure. The back passage is
 closed and the end of the gut is attached to an
 opening in the wall of the tummy. A bag is attached
 to the opening. (to which / where)

4 It's a type of shock. It happens when the volume of
 blood in the body decreases. (which / who)

5 Oliguria is a condition. An abnormally small amount
 of urine is produced. (where / that)

6 It's an operation. The appendix is removed. There
 is colicky pain in the centre of the tummy followed
 by vomiting and then a shift of the pain to the right
 iliac fossa. (where / when)

» Go to **Grammar reference** p 124

Patient care

1 Putting yourself in the patient's shoes, what would you
 ask in response to the explanations in *Language spot*?

2 Match these responses to the explanations 1–6 in
 Language spot.
 a Will it pass?
 b Are there complications if it is removed?
 c Will that get rid of the cancer, then?
 d But will it be permanent?
 e Does that mean it will be difficult to see?
 f Can you get it back to normal?

3 Take turns explaining the terms in *Language spot* and
 responding using the phrases in **2**, then developing the
 conversation in your own way.

Project

1 Work in groups. Using your own knowledge, describe
 how pain is managed after an operation.

2 Find out about the organizations and sites below and
 what they do. Do they give any advice about pain
 management after operations?
 • colostomy – colostomyassociation.org.uk
 • kidney / kidney stones – kidney.org, medlineplus.gov
 • hysterectomy – hysterectomy-association.org.uk
 • mastectomy – medlineplus.gov
 • tonsillectomy – patient.co.uk
 • hernia – hernia.org

3 In groups, discuss different reactions to pain. How do
 people measure pain?

4 Check your answers about pain in the *Oxford Textbook
 of Palliative Medicine*, 3rd edition, (Doyle et al, 2005,
 OUP). Also look at pages 172–181 of the *Oxford Handbook
 of Palliative Care* (Watson et al, 2005, OUP).

5 Work in pairs. Choose a procedure. Take turns being the
 doctor talking to the patient about post-operative pain.
 USEFUL EXPRESSIONS
 sore   hurt   discomfort

Speaking

1 Work in groups. Decide how you would explain to a patient that he is going to need a permanent colostomy after removal of the part of the bowel. Discuss what information a patient would want to know in order to give consent for the operation, especially about the future, e.g. pain management. Use the questions in **2** in *Listening 1* as a guide.

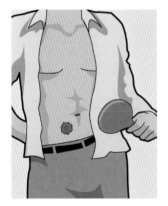 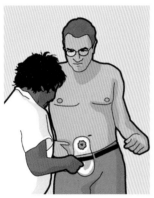 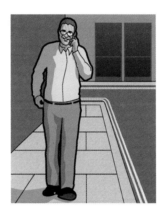 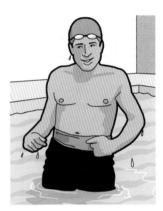

2 Work with a partner from another group. Decide on a name, age, and sex for the patient. Take turns role-playing explaining the operation to the patient and obtaining consent. If you are not happy with the explanation, decline to give consent.

3 When you have finished, as a whole class discuss any medical problems or queries that arose during the role-play.

4 In exam situations, you are faced with role-plays which you need to do without any preparation. Look at this role-play scenario by yourself.

> Mr Cordobes, a 30-year-old man, has a ten-year-old son who has been involved in a car accident. The child's spleen has been damaged and his femur has been fractured. His spleen is so badly damaged that it needs to be removed. You have to tell the patient's father and explain the procedure to him. What would you say?

USEFUL EXPRESSIONS
emergency operation
no choice
We can boost his immune system starting now until he's an adult.
It is possible to live without the spleen.

5 You have five minutes to think about the scenario by yourself, focusing on both the doctor's and the patient's roles. Note in exam situations you will usually have only one minute to walk between stations, read, and prepare to role-play the scenario.

6 Two volunteers role-play the scenario in front of the class. Students sit around so that they can see both the doctor and the patient. The doctors who are watching use the speaking checklist on page 117 to choose a criterion each to assess the performance. Agree all the criteria beforehand. Some students should also observe the doctor to see if their performance is sympathetic / empathetic. Students take turns role-playing and giving feedback. The feedback should be constructive.

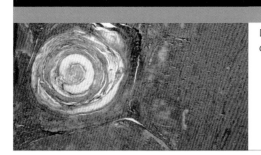

Dermoid ovarian cyst

Reading

1 Skim this summary text. What do you think it is describing?

The majority of cysts in the ovaries are harmless and
¹_____, but some trigger changes in the
²_____ as well as in the nature of the periods.
Cysts can also become so big that they cause urine
problems or make people ³_____. Despite being
generally harmless, some can turn to ⁴_____.

⁵_____ is frequently down to luck, so if you
have any symptoms that ⁶_____that you
have an ovarian cyst, an internal examination may be
performed by your doctor. Treatment is ⁷_____
on various factors like age and the cyst size.

2 Read the text below. Complete the summary in 1 using
the correct form of a word from the text.

What are the symptoms, problems, and possible complications?

Most ovarian cysts are small, benign (non-cancerous), and cause no symptoms. Some ovarian cysts cause problems which may include one or more of the following:

- Pain or discomfort in the lower abdomen. The pain may be constant or intermittent. Pain may only occur when you have sex.
- Periods sometimes become irregular, or may become heavier or lighter than usual.
- Sometimes a cyst may bleed into itself or burst. This can cause a sudden severe pain in the lower abdomen.
- Occasionally, a cyst which is growing on a stalk from an ovary may twist the stalk on itself (a 'torsion'). This stops the blood flowing through the stalk to the cyst and causes the cyst to lose its blood supply. This can cause sudden severe pain in the lower abdomen.
- Large cysts can cause your abdomen to swell or press on nearby structures. For example, they may press on the bladder or rectum which may cause urinary symptoms or constipation.

- Although most cysts are benign, some types have a risk of becoming cancerous.
- Rarely, some ovarian cysts make abnormal amounts of female (or male) hormones which can cause unusual symptoms.

How is an ovarian cyst diagnosed?

As most ovarian cysts cause no symptoms, many cysts are diagnosed by chance. For example, during a routine examination, or if you have an ultrasound scan for another reason. If you have symptoms suggestive of an ovarian cyst, your doctor may examine your abdomen and perform a vaginal (internal) examination. He or she may be able to feel an abnormal swelling which may be a cyst.

An ultrasound scan can confirm an ovarian cyst. An ultrasound scan is a safe and painless test which uses sound waves to create images of organs and structures inside your body. The probe of the scanner may be placed on your abdomen to scan the ovaries. A small probe is also often placed inside the vagina to scan the ovaries to obtain more detailed images. Your doctor may also take a sample of blood.

What is the treatment for ovarian cysts?

Your specialist will advise on the best course of action. This depends on factors

such as your age, whether you are past the menopause, the appearance and size of the cyst from the ultrasound scan, and whether you have symptoms.

Observation

Many small ovarian cysts will resolve and disappear over a few months. You may be advised to have a repeat ultrasound scan in a month or so. If the cyst goes away, then no further action is needed.

Operation

Removal of an ovarian cyst may be advised, especially if you have symptoms or if the cyst is large. Sometimes the specialist may want to remove it to determine exactly which type of cyst it is and make sure there are no cancer cells in it. Most smaller cysts can be removed by laparoscopic ('keyhole') surgery. Some cysts require a more traditional style of operation.

The type of the operation depends on factors such as the type of cyst, your age, and whether cancer is suspected or ruled out. In some cases, just the cyst is removed and the ovary tissue preserved. In some cases, the ovary is also removed, and sometimes other nearby structures such as the uterus and the other ovary. Your specialist will advise on the options for your individual situation.

3 Match the two parts of the sentences below.

1 Many small cysts simply	a leave the ovary tissue.
2 Size and symptoms sometimes	b ascertain cyst type.
3 Cyst removal may be done to	c dictate the surgical removal of ovarian cysts.
4 Sometimes it is possible to	d go away in a matter of months

4 Work in groups. Talk about the first time you were involved in an operation and your reaction(s).

Listening 2

Getting into conversations

1 🎧 Listen to the five short conversations and decide what each one is about. Time how long it takes you to work out what is happening and put your hand up when you have worked it out, but do not interrupt the playing of the recording.

2 🎧 Listen again and match the five conversations with these descriptions.

a _____ Anaesthetic assessment

b _____ Worried about recurrence of a problem

c _____ Postponement

d _____ Awake in day surgery

e _____ Refusing consent

3 🎧 Listen again. Work in pairs. One partner concentrates on the patient and the other on the doctor. Write down how the patient puts pressure on the doctor and how the doctor resists pressure from the patient. Compare your answers with another pair.

4 Work in pairs. Create a scenario around one of the conversations, giving the patient a name, age, and so on. Take turns role-playing the situations and then developing them in your own way. For example, for extract 5, you could take a pre-operative assessment, asking about the drug and family history.

Vocabulary

Technical vocabulary

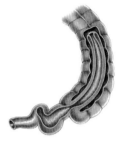

1 Work in pairs. Describe the condition shown in the diagram. Can it occur at any age?

2 Work in groups. Complete the sentences. If necessary look at the words in the upside-down box below.

1 The small bowel _____ as if it were swallowing itself by invagination.

2 The patient presents with episodic intermittent _____ crying and drawing his legs up.

3 The child may pass blood per _____ (like redcurrant jam or merely flecks – late stage).

4 A sausage-shaped _____ may be felt.

5 The child may be _____ and moribund.

6 The least _____ approach is ultrasound with reduction by air enema (preferred to barium).

7 Pneumatic _____, where a balloon catheter is passed PR under radiographic control, is another option that is effective in up to 80% of cases.

8 There may be right lower quadrant _____ ± perforation on plain abdominal film.

9 If reduction by enema fails, reduction at laparoscopy or _____ is needed.

10 Any necrotic bowel should be _____.

		telescopes	shocked
	rectum	reduction	opacity
inconsolable	invasive	laparotomy	mass
	mass	laparotomy	resected

3 Check with other groups for help with sentences you cannot complete.

4 Work in pairs. Choose a sentence from 2 for your partner to explain to you what it means in lay terms. Use your own experience if possible.

USEFUL EXPRESSIONS
get rid of   doesn't work   fold inside itself
what we're going to need to do   remove

Speaking

1 Work in groups. Look at the scenario below. Decide what the patient is likely to be concerned about, for example, the recurrence of the cysts, whether they are cancerous, what caused them, why it happened to her, the length of time off work. What is she likely to say and what would be your reply?

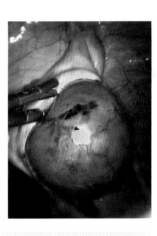

> Miss Tanaka, who is 22 years old, has been admitted to hospital after being diagnosed as having a right ovarian cyst. A laparotomy is going to be performed and she has to stay in hospital for four days and subsequently stay at home for six weeks. Explain the situation to her. Note that a sub-cuticle suture is going to be used for skin repair.

2 Decide how you are going to explain what a cyst is, where it is, what is going to be removed, and what is going to be done with the removed cyst. Then decide how to describe the sub-cuticle suture, and finally when to ask the patient to sign the consent form.

3 Take turns role-playing the scenario in the 'goldfish bowl' setting described in Unit 5. This time, however, the doctor or the patient may interrupt the role-play to ask questions or clarify specific details. Limit each interruption to a maximum of two minutes.

4 Give feedback to the doctor and the patient using the speaking checklist on page 117.

5 When two or three pairs have done the role-play, work on your own. In two minutes, prepare what you would say to the patient for the scenario below and repeat steps 3 and 4 above.

> Mrs Brodie's eight-month-old baby has been crying / screaming for the past eight hours, i.e. all night. The findings show the baby is suffering from intussusception. Explain to the mother what it is and how it will be treated.

Project

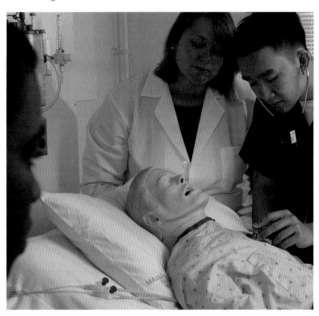

1 Use these references to find out what you can about OSCE exams, especially for the PLAB, USMLE, and fellowship exams for the Royal Colleges in the UK:
   - www.gmc.org
   - For DOPS (directly observed procedural skills) see the Royal College – www.rcplondon.ac.uk
   - USMLE – www.usmle.org

2 How many stations are there in an OSCE and how long does a station last?

3 Which of the following stations are normally found in an OSCE?
   - ☐ Taking blood pressure
   - ☐ Doing CPR
   - ☐ Giving a presentation
   - ☐ Explaining procedures to a patient
   - ☐ Taking a case history
   - ☐ Reciting medical detail
   - ☐ Dealing with difficult situations
   - ☐ Suturing
   - ☐ Using manikins for clinical examinations

Writing

Describing a complicated operation

1 Work in pairs. Describe a complicated operation which you have been involved in, focusing on *pre-operative visit, assessment by the anaesthetist, the day of the operation*, and *post-operative care*, including *pain management*. Mention anything that went particularly well, anything that could have gone better, and what you would have done differently.

2 Work on your own. Write a description of no more than 200 words, using the phrases in italics in **1** as a step-by-step guide.

USEFUL EXPRESSIONS
... an operation where ...
Moreover, ... / Furthermore, ...
The benefit of ... was ...
The main thing I learnt from this was ...
... worked well / ... went smoothly / What could have gone better was ...

3 Work in pairs. Check for mistakes. Remember not to copy each other's writing and to maintain anonymity and confidentiality.

4 Give your description to another partner to read. Ask each other questions about the description: *Why did you ...? What factors made ...? Could you have ...?*

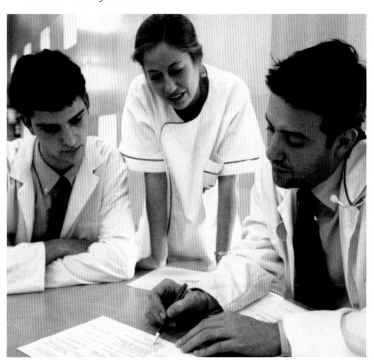

Key words

Adjective
inconsolable

Nouns
consent
day-case surgery
herniorrhaphy
intussusception
laparotomy
perforated appendix
reduction

Verbs
glove
gown
resect
scrub up
telescope

Prefixes
col(on)-
cysto-
hystero-
laparo-
masto- / mammo-
nephro-

Useful reference

Oxford Handbook of Clinical Surgery
3rd edition, McLatchie et al (eds),
ISBN 978-019-856825-4

9 Cardiology

Check up

1 Work in pairs. Describe the pictures.

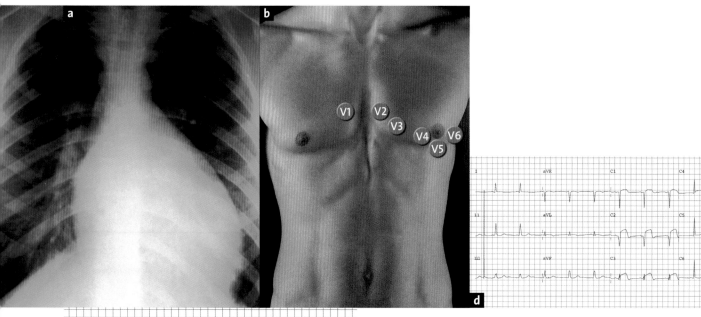

2 Match these captions to the ECGs in **1**.
- Acute anterior myocardial infarction
- Complete heart block

3 Look at these statistics for the UK taken from the *Oxford Handbook of General Practice*. Is the incidence of heart disease higher or lower in your country? Why?

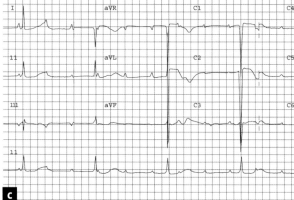

> Coronary heart disease (CHD) is the most common cause of death in the UK (1:4 deaths). Mortality is falling, but morbidity is rising.

Listening 1

A heart condition

1 🎧 Listen to Mr Lawson's wife talking to the doctor in A&E. What do you think the patient's condition is? Why?

2 Describe the doctor's manner and the mood of the patient's wife. Give reasons.

3 🎧 Listen again and write down notes on what is said about
   1 the GTN spray
   2 the time when the pain started
   3 thrombolysis
   4 prognosis.

4 🎧 Work in groups. Compare your notes and listen again. Discuss the possible differential diagnosis of the patient's condition.

5 Choose one member to report back to the whole class.

6 Work in pairs. Take turns role-playing the conversation between a patient's spouse and a doctor with the same presentation as in **1**.

Vocabulary

Avoidance of technical terms

1 In these sentences, the speaker is trying to avoid using one of the technical words or phrases in the list below. Match each word to a sentence.

a	hypokalaemia	f	line
b	titrate to effect	g	secure venous access
c	diuretic	h	reperfuse
d	contraindication	i	thrombolysis
e	arrhythmia	j	tolerate

1 If we can, we give him a drug to dissolve any clots, then we increase his chances of getting better.
2 My heart is not beating in a normal rhythm.
3 There are several reasons why this drug should not be used.
4 You have no side effects with this drug.
5 We're going to give you something to help reduce the swelling in your ankles.
6 As soon as the patient is brought in, we need to get into a vein.
7 We'll increase the painkiller by the same amount each time until it kicks in.
8 This drug will get the blood flowing back again through the heart.
9 If this doesn't work, we'll move onto the next stage of treatment.
10 You've got very low levels of potassium.

2 Work in groups. Choose a drug that is recommended for use in thrombolysis or treating myocardial infarction or hypertension (e.g. ace inhibitor, a diuretic, (simva) statin, aspirin.) Discuss your own experience of prescribing the drug.

● Language spot

The future

1 Work in pairs. What tenses are used in these sentences?

1 The ward round starts at 10, so we have half an hour.
2 She normally stops at 12, but today, I think she'll have finished her rounds well before 11.30.
3 The ward round is finishing at 12 noon.
4 So we'll definitely be sitting in the canteen at 1.10.
5 We'll have been working for 12 hours by 1.00 this afternoon.

2 Work in pairs. Read all the sentences 1–6 below, then match them with the relevant points or periods on the diagram.

A	B	C	D	E	F		G	H
9 a.m.	**10** a.m.	**11** a.m.	**12** noon	**1** p.m.	**2** p.m.		**6** p.m.	**7** p.m.

(Now)

1 We'll have had eight hours on duty by the end of the day.
2 We're having an hour for lunch.
3 We'll have just finished lunch by the time the consultant arrives for her ward rounds.
4 The weekly presentation, which will last two hours, will end just before lunch.
5 Dr Ian Garfield will be starting the presentation as soon as he arrives.
6 The shift today starts at 10.00 with a presentation.

3 Work in pairs. Put the verbs in brackets into the correct future form in the active or passive.

1 If his progress so far is anything to go by, he _____ (be) up and about in a few days.
2 He _____ (send) home this Saturday.
3 She _____ (soon move) out of intensive care.
4 That means in ten minutes, it _____ (be) roughly 60 minutes since the pain first came on.
5 He _____ (walk) around without any problem in a matter of days.
6 _____ (he be able) to go into a rehabilitation unit before he comes out?
7 What _____ (he have) to eat by the time I get there today?
8 The consultant _____ (come) round at about 1.00 p.m., so we _____ (see) him then.

4 Work in pairs. Prepare three or four questions about what you will have done, are planning to do, will be doing, and will do today. Give your questions to your partner and then ask each other the questions.

>> Go to **Grammar reference** p 124

Pronunciation

Speaking at natural speed

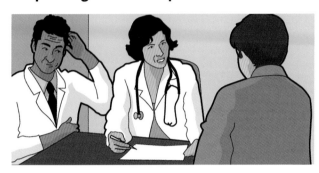

When people speak at natural speed, it is possible to catch the gist of what they say, but sometimes the exact words can be difficult to work out.

1 🎧 Listen and complete the sentences. Note that contractions are used.

1 _____ theatre for over three hours in a few minutes' time.

2 Dr Nur _____ his clinic till 2.00 p.m.

3 _____ in no time.

4 All being well, _____ home by the weekend.

5 The operation _____ for 5.00 this afternoon.

6 _____ the veins on the right leg stripped this afternoon, am I right?

7 The doctor said _____ a general anaesthetic.

8 _____ to the clinic off and on for the past three years.

2 Work in pairs. Compare your answers.

3 🎧 Listen again. Check your answers.

4 🎧 Listen again. In each sentence, <u><u>double underline</u></u> the nucleus. <u>Single underline</u> the secondary stresses.

5 Work in pairs. Take turns saying only the stressed words in each sentence. Then say the whole sentence using the stressed words to give you the rhythm.

Patient care

1 Work in pairs. How would you respond to the statements below, made by the spouse of a patient who has just been brought into A&E suffering from a heart attack?

1 He's been in the theatre for ages now.

2 Things are looking bad, aren't they?

3 Will he be OK?

4 He looks rather well.

5 I'm a bit anxious about what'll happen with the procedure you described.

6 How long's he going to be in here?

7 He thinks he's going to die, doctor.

2 Compare your statements with other students. Then discuss them with the class.

3 Work in pairs. What type of word is missing in the blank spaces (noun, verb, etc.)? Complete the responses below with one word.

a Oh. It's only a _____ of days now. In fact, he'll be seeing the consultant tomorrow morning and if he's happy, you can …

b Yes, he does. And if _____ goes according to plan, this time next week I expect he'll be sitting at home with you.

c It's not _____ to feel this, but you got him here quickly, which'll _____ help him.

d It's actually not as bad as it seems. The machines and tubes, I'm _____, don't make things look good, but they're there to help him. He'll be like this for a little _____ and then …

e Yes. We expect he'll be ready to leave in a couple of days. It's the anaesthetic and the painkillers; they're making him a bit confused, but that'll soon _____ off.

f It always seems longer when you're sitting waiting. I'm sure he'll be _____ shortly; in fact, here's the nurse now.

g It's only _____ to feel worried; everybody would be, but I can assure you it'll help him.

4 Match each response a–g to a statement in 1.

5 Work in pairs. Take turns saying the statements in 1 to each other and responding in your own way.

Remember the mnemonic **SOCRATES** for questions related to pain.

Dialogue can transform a symptom from airy nothingness to a fact.

Dialogue-transformed symptoms explain one of the junior doctor's main vexations: when patients retell symptoms to a consultant in the light of day they bear no resemblance to what you originally heard. But do not be vexed: your dialogue may have helped the patient more than any ward round.

– Oxford Handbook of Clinical Medicine

Signs and symptoms

Competition

1 Work in groups. Using your own experience, decide what conditions the following signs and symptoms represent. Compete to see which group finishes with all the correct answers first.

1 Symptoms: dyspnoea, cough productive of frothy pink sputum, palpitations (often associated with atrial fibrillation and resultant emboli)
Signs: palmar erythema, malar flush, tapping apex beat, left parasternal heave, loud S1, mid-diastolic murmur + opening snap.

2 Symptoms: shortness of breath and breathing worse on lying flat
Signs: collapsing pulse, sustained apex beat displaced to the left, left parasternal heave, soft S1, loud S2 (pulmonary component), pansystolic murmur heard at the apex and radiating to the left axilla + mid-systolic click, 3rd heart sound.

3 Symptoms: calf pain, swelling and loss of use
Signs: warm, tense, swollen limb, erythema, dilated superficial veins, cyanosis. There may be palpable thrombus in the deep veins. Often pain on palpating the calf.

4 Symptoms: constant retrosternal 'soreness', worse on inspiration (pleuritic), relieved slightly by sitting forwards, not related to movement or exertion
Signs: If chronic, constrictive, may cause Kussmaul's sign, impalpable apex beat, S3, hepatomegaly, splenomegaly, ascites (pseudo-cirrhosis).

4 pericarditis
3 deep vein thrombosis (DVT)
2 mitral regurgitation
1 mitral stenosis

2 Work in groups. Choose one of the conditions in 1. Present the details to the rest of the class. You may do this as a formal PowerPoint presentation with a question and answer session at the end, or informally on behalf of your groups with questions at the end.

Project

1 Work in groups. Make a list of cardiac risk factors. Search for information at www.americanheart.org.

Speaking

1 Work in groups of four. Make a list of questions you would ask the patient in the scenario below. Think about how the patient would feel, what his / her anxieties might be, and how you differentiate the pain from *angina pectoris*.

Mr Gregory, a 57-year-old patient, presents with a severe retrosternal burning pain which the patient is convinced is connected with the heart. The pain comes after eating and drinking alcohol and there is a history of dyspepsia. The pain is relieved by GTN spray, but only after about twenty minutes. Take the history and reassure the patient that the pain is not connected with his heart, but is oesophageal spasm.

2 Take turns role-playing taking the history and reassuring the patient. During each role-play, the two other students use the checklist on page 117 to monitor the performance of the patient and the doctor, who choose at least two criteria to be assessed on: *asking questions, empathy / sympathy, reassurance, prognosis, and clarity of pronunciation.*

3 One of the monitoring doctors times the role-play: a maximum of five minutes.

4 The doctor and the patient each give feedback about themselves and each other. The monitors also give feedback. Then the roles are rotated to allow each group member a chance to role-play the doctor.

5 One pair of students (or more) volunteers to role-play the scenario while the rest of the class watches and gives feedback.

6 Student A, go to page 114. Student B, go to page 115. Student B, take the history from student A and reassure the patient and vice versa. At the relevant point the patient gives the doctor the ECG.

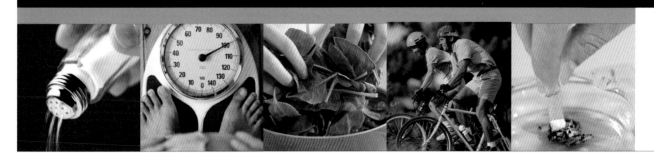

Reading

1 Work in pairs. Discuss these questions.
1 What do you know about hypertension?
2 What are the causes? What is the usual presentation?
3 Have you treated a patient with hypertension? Was it drug or non-drug treatment?

2 Find these items in the text.
1 a definition
2 an effect of treatment
3 prevalence of high BP
4 precipitating factors / aetiology of the high BP
5 a connection with other illnesses

High Blood Pressure – Hypertension

Hypertension (HT) is commonly called high blood pressure, nowadays (2005 on) defined as above 140/85 mm Hg; or if one is diabetic, over 135/80. About 38% of UK adults have hypertension. Advice and treatment includes exercise, lifestyle changes, and / or diet changes, as well as drugs.

Possibly as many as 16 million UK people have high blood pressure, and the proportion of the population is slowly increasing over the years. About 5% have an obvious underlying cause such as kidney disease. Most of the rest have no single obvious cause. Some have a genetic component, with hypertension tending to run in families. In addition there are environmental and lifestyle factors. The most important causes are being obese, smoking, too much alcohol, too much salt, stress, lack of exercise, poor diet, too little potassium, and family history of relatives with hypertension. Oily fish with omega-3 fatty acids is protective against high blood pressure and heart disease.

Hypertension – why worry if you feel OK?

High blood pressure does not necessarily make someone feel unwell; however, if untreated it tends to cause damage to blood vessels and the heart. The link between hypertension and coronary heart disease and stroke is very well established.

Correct treatment of hypertension reduces the risk of a heart attack by about 20% and reduces the risk of stroke by about 40%. Here risk is based on the observed reduced occurrences in treated past patients. The purpose of treating hypertension is to prevent this damage to blood vessels and the heart from occurring and so help to prevent these illnesses. Most people with hypertension need tablets to lower their blood pressure. Usually, they need to continue them for life. These tablets are very successful at preventing heart attacks and strokes and have very few side effects.

Five self-help measures are suggested:

◾ Avoid being overweight.

◾ Reduce salt intake.

◾ Keep alcohol down.

◾ Exercise can reduce your blood pressure and help to keep your weight down. Start slowly and build up. Walking is excellent. Aim for 20 to 30 minutes' activity at least three times a week. Or even better, walk for half an hour five times per week, which is better than more intense exercise for a shorter time.

◾ Don't smoke.

3 Complete these notes using a word or a number from the text.

- HT for diabetic patients[1]_____
- Modifications to [2]_____ plus possibly diet and medication recommended
- For [3]_____ people not just one cause
- [4]_____ fatty acids help against high blood pressure and heart disease
- Connection with coronary heart disease and stroke [5]_____

4 Discuss in groups:
- How common is hypertension in your country or where you work?
- What measures are being taken to reduce it?
- Are they effective? Give reasons and examples.

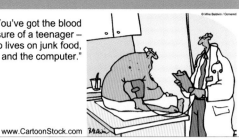

"You've got the blood pressure of a teenager – who lives on junk food, TV and the computer."

www.CartoonStock.com

Listening 2

Advice about lifestyle changes

1 🎧 Listen. Write down as many details as you can about the patient. Then compare your details in groups of four.

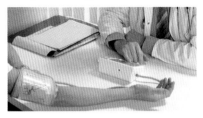

2 Before you listen again, can you answer any of the questions below from the information you have?
1 What evidence can you find of the doctor's good bedside manner?
2 What evidence can you find of the patient's cooperative manner?
3 How does the doctor seek to involve the patient in lifestyle changes?
4 How does the doctor make a suggestion about lifestyle changes?
5 How does the doctor reassure the patient of the effect of the lifestyle change suggested?

3 🎧 Listen again. Answer the questions.

4 What other lifestyle changes could the doctor encourage this patient to make? How else could the doctor phrase his suggestions?

Patient care

When patients are hypertensive, they may have no symptoms. It is therefore not always easy for them to accept or follow any therapy or even remember to keep to it. You, therefore, need to be able to give patients advice and information in a way that fits the situation and doesn't put them off.

Look at the following examples:

Stop smoking.

The imperative here is inappropriate for giving patients advice about lifestyle changes.

Have you thought about taking this tablet once a day after meals?

The suggestion here doesn't work because you want to direct the patient. It would be better to say: *You take / Take this tablet ... or You'll need to take this tablet once a day after meals.*

1 Work in groups. Look at these statements. Where and when can you say them without annoying a patient? Which are appropriate for making suggestions to patients about changing their lifestyle to reduce the risk of future heart attack? Give reasons.

1 You'll need to stop smoking from now on.
2 You could stop driving for a while, say six weeks.
3 Have you ever tried to do any kind of sport?
4 Don't take any alcohol.
5 I'd strongly advise you to take the medication.
6 It's better for you if you avoid salt.
7 You need to make sure you take this regularly.
8 You might want to take this medication from now on.
9 You shouldn't eat fatty food like sweets and cakes.
10 Try and give up smoking if you can.
11 You take this one once a day, preferably in the evening.
12 You need to come back and see me after one month.

2 Work in pairs. Write at least three sentences giving advice about these topics.

1 caffeine and caffeine-rich products
2 relaxation / stress management
3 dynamic exercise – walking, swimming, cycling
4 salt intake
5 fruit and fibre

3 Work in pairs. Using the notes you made in *Listening 2*, take turns role-playing the conversation between Mary and her GP. Continue giving advice to Mary about changes to lifestyle. Emphasize the benefits the changes will bring.

USEFUL EXPRESSIONS
If you ...
It'll make you ...
You'll soon notice the difference.
It'll reduce ...
All being well, you'll have ...

Cardiovascular disease is estimated to cost the EU economy €192 billion a year. 57% is due to direct health care costs, 21% to productivity losses and 22% to the informal care of people with CVD.

Costs vary hugely between EU member states – per capita annually, Bulgaria costs under €60 but Germany and the UK cost over €600.

– *European Heart Network*

Speaking

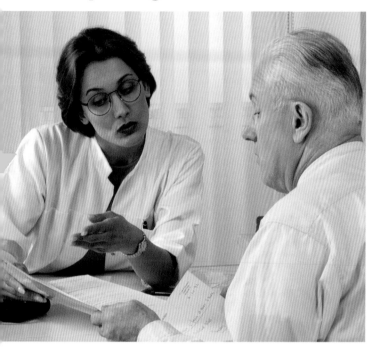

1 Work in pairs. Take turns talking to a 65-year-old, Vincent Fournier, who presents with hypertension, about the medication he needs to take.

Check for any contraindications.

Explain:
- how to take the medication
- when to take it
- the benefits of taking it
- any side effects.

Arrange for follow-up in one month's time.

2 Two students volunteer to role-play the part of the doctor and the patient in the scenario below in front of the class. Use the Checklist on page 117 to give feedback using the following two criteria: ability to encourage the patient and spontaneity.

A 55-year-old patient, Mr(s) Slater, has high cholesterol. Give advice about non-drug therapy for high cholesterol with written instructions and / or drug therapy with benefits and side effects.

3 Give feedback. Remember to be constructive.

Project

1 Work in groups. Search for information on the web or in books or pool your own experience. Each group should research a different subject from:

1 drug treatment for hypertension
2 prescribing statins for hypercholesterolaemia, especially any contraindications and side effects
3 non-drug therapy for cholesterol

2 Type in the words *statin, hypertension, cholesterol* on the internet or check these sources.
- www.bhsoc.org
- www.nice.org.uk
- www.patient.co.uk
- www.yourtotalhealth.ivillage.com
- www.bhf.org.uk

Also check the Oxford Handbook of General Practice, 2nd edition pages 324–5

3 Select which information to talk about and share the information with the class.

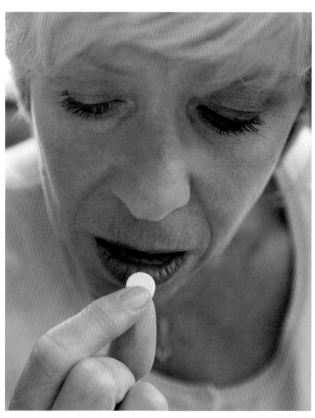

Writing

Difficulties in persuasion

1 Work in pairs. Make a list of the difficulties doctors face trying to persuade patients of the need to take medication. Explain the difficulties, giving examples from your own experience. Remember to maintain confidentiality.

2 Compare your list with other students in the class and add to your own list.

3 Work on your own. Write between 200 and 250 words explaining the difficulties you listed in **1**. Use the useful expressions and suggested plan to guide you as you write your answer.

USEFUL EXPRESSIONS
main obstacles
problems faced by doctors
First of all / second(ly) / third(ly)
In addition, / furthermore / similarly
In conclusion, / as we have seen,

Introduction: an overview or example of the topic

The main barrier ...

Another difficulty ...

... can also effect patient's compliance.

Conclusion or summary

Checklist

Assess your progress in this unit.
Tick (✓) the statements which are true.

I can understand and use technical and non-technical terms

I can talk about the future and reassure patients about the prognosis

I can talk about heart disease

I can talk about signs and symptoms

I can understand people speaking at natural speed

Key words

Adjectives
frothy

Nouns
arrhythmia
atrial fibrillation
cholesterol
contraindication
diuretic
DVT
dynamic exercise
hypertension
lifestyle
line
mitral stenosis
morbidity
mortality
pericarditis
SOCRATES
statin
thrombolysis

Verb
tolerate

Useful reference

Oxford Handbook of Clinical Medicine
7th edition, Longmore et al,
ISBN 978-0-19-856837-7

10 Respiratory medicine

Check up

1 Work in groups. Describe the photos. What is the link between the photos? Give an example relating to each photo.

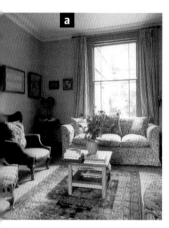
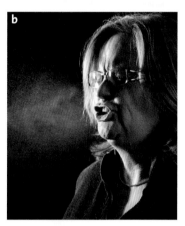
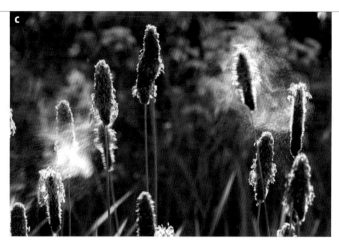
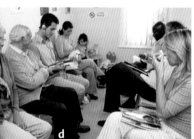
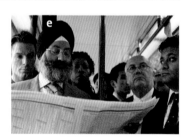
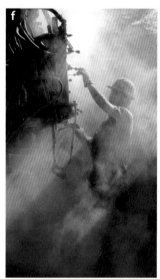

2 Work in groups. Describe interesting presentations involving respiratory medicine that you dealt with successfully. Describe how you might improve your performance if you were to see the same case again.

3 What is the definition of asthma? What symptoms would you expect to see?

4 Asthma affects 5–8% of the population in the UK. What is the percentage in your country? Is it increasing or decreasing? What are the causes in your country?

Vocabulary

Coughs

1 Choose the adjective that best fits the diagnosis in italics in each case.

1 Laryngitis: I've got this really bad cough and my voice is *high-pitched / hoarse / smooth*.
2 Tracheitis: I've got a dry cough and it's *slightly painful / painless / really painful*.
3 Pleurisy: my chest really hurts when I cough. I get this *stabbing / dull / sharp* pain right here in the chest when I cough.
4 Post-nasal drip: I've not got any pain or anything; just a dry, *barking / tickly / painful* cough. I'm always trying to clear my throat at night.
5 Asthma: I've been getting this *wheezy / tickly / painful* cough after doing exercise and sometimes in the morning.
6 Oesophageal reflux: first thing in the morning I get this *dry / tickly / hollow* cough and it often makes me feel sick.
7 Epiglottis: she's really poorly with this terrible *tickly / barking / dry* cough.
8 Laryngeal nerve palsy: the cough sounds really *barking / hoarse / hollow*.
9 Bronchitis: he's had this *productive / mild / hollow* cough for days now with some fever but no breathlessness.

2 🎧 Listen and identify the coughs which you hear 1–5 as *wheezy, hoarse, productive, barking, dry*. Check your answers with a partner.

In this unit
- language for cough and sputum
- explaining investigations
- using *a / an*, *the*, and zero article
- checking the patient understands devices
- describing data

3 Work in pairs. Take turns asking a patient to describe one of the coughs in **2** and then develop the conversation using your own knowledge.

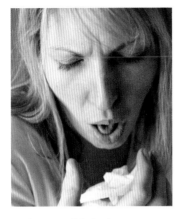

Listening 1

Signs and symptoms

1 Work in pairs. Decide what the most likely diagnosis is of a patient who presents with recurrent episodes of bronchitis several years prior to presentation with these signs and symptoms:

Signs
1 coarse inspiratory and expiratory crackles on auscultation
2 airflow obstruction with wheeze

Symptoms
1 cough
2 chronic sputum production (typically tenacious, purulent, and daily)
3 intermittent haemoptyses
4 breathlessness
5 intermittent pleuritic pain (usually in association with infections)
6 lethargy / malaise

2 🎧 Work in pairs. Listen to the conversation between Dr Zoltan and Mrs Fitzgerald, who is not asthmatic and is a non-smoker. Student A, listen to the questions the doctor asks and write them down in note form. Student B, write down what the patient says.

3 Using the doctor's questions as a guide, explain what the patient says and decide on a possible diagnosis. Is it the same as in **1** above? If not, why not?

Vocabulary

Nature of the sputum

1 Cover the causes a–h in the right hand column with your hand and use your own knowledge to diagnose the cause of the sputum 1–8.

Nature of sputum	Causes
1 white / grey	a bronchiectasis / abscesses
2 green / yellow	
3 green and offensive	b congestive cardiac failure
4 sticky, rusty	c asthma / smoking
5 frothy, pink	d severe bronchiectasis
6 separates to three layers	e bronchitis / bronchiectasis
7 very sticky, often green	f asthma
8 sticky, with plugs	g allergic aspergillosis
	h lobar pneumonia

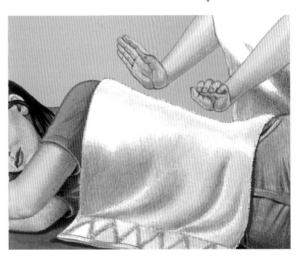

2 Match the nature of the sputum to the causes in **1**.

3 Apart from the nature of the sputum, what investigations / tests would you do to establish the causes in a–h?

4 Work in pairs. Choose one of the conditions in **1**. Then take turns taking the history from each other.

5 Work in pairs. Choose several of the conditions a –h. Explain to the patient what you think the diagnosis might be and what tests you are going to do.

afferent (adj) carrying or directing something towards a body part
cessation (n) stopping
lodged (adj) stuck
OSA Obstructive Sleep Apnoea
COPD Chronic Obstructive Pulmonary Disease

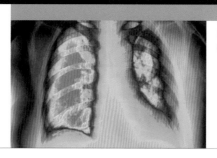

Pulmonary embolism

● Language spot
The definite and indefinite article

1 Work in pairs. Complete the sentences using *the, a, an*, or zero article (0).

1 _____ breathlessness refers to _____ abnormal and uncomfortable awareness of breathing. Its physiological mechanisms are poorly understood; _____ possible afferent sources for _____ sensation include _____ receptors in _____ respiratory muscles. All patients need _____ full history and examination.

2 _____ smoking is _____ main cause of _____ chronic obstructive pulmonary disease and lung cancer. _____ NHS spends £1.7 billion per year caring for people with _____ smoking-related conditions. Government targets have been set to reduce _____ number of smokers in _____ UK, and health authorities have been allocated funding for _____ smoking cessation services.

2 In the sentences below, find the four extra definite articles.

1 The mortality for patients with the pneumonia who are managed in the community is less than 1%, but one in four patients with pneumonia is admitted to hospital and mortality for those admitted is around 9%.

2 TB is spread by the airborne droplets containing mycobacterium tuberculosis (MTB). Droplets can remain airborne for hours after the expectoration because of their small size. Infectious droplets are inhaled and become lodged in the distal airways.

3 Pulmonary embolism is a clinically significant obstruction of part or all of the pulmonary vascular tree, usually caused by the thrombus from a different site.

3 In the sentences below, put the words in italics in the correct order to complete the texts. Pay particular attention to the articles.

1 *The / majority / chest / patients / of / with / pain / referred / to / have / acute / either / pleuritic / the / respiratory / team / well-localized / pain / pain / or / persistent.*

2 Not all patients need treatment. *evidence / significant / treatment / the / for / on / benefits / symptoms / rests, / which / drive / treatment*, rather than the degree of OSA on a sleep study. *decisions / require / a / dialogue / treatment / close / between / patient / physician / and.*

3 In addition to supportive care, antiviral treatment of pneumonia with amantidine or rimantidine may shorten *the / an / of / illness / if / started / duration / of / symptom / within / hours / 48 / onset.*

>> Go to **Grammar reference** p 125

Listening 2
Mistake recognition

1 🎧 Listen to the recording of five pairs of statements. Decide in which statement (a or b) the use of the articles is correct.

2 🎧 Check your answers with a partner and listen again.

3 🎧 Work in pairs. Listen to sentences 1–7 in turn and decide together whether the articles in each sentence are correct. Check your answers with another pair.

4 🎧 Listen again and check your answers.

Speaking

Work in pairs. Rank these causes of breathlessness in order of speed of onset: *Instantaneous, Acute* (minutes–hours), *Subacute* (days), *Chronic* (months–years). Check your answers with another pair.

pleural effusion   pneumothorax
fibrotic lung disease   exacerbations of asthma
COPD   pulmonary embolism
asbestosis

TB tuberculosis
resolve (v) disappear

Signs and symptoms

Lung conditions

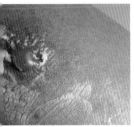
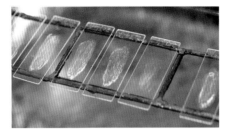

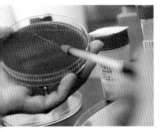
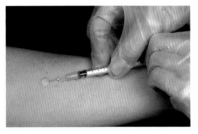

1 Work in pairs. Choose one of these clinical conditions and symptoms 1–6. What questions would you ask to reach a possible diagnosis?

1 Pneumonia
fever, rigors malaise, anorexia, dyspnoea, cough, purulent sputum, haemoptysis, and pleuritic pain

2 TB
productive cough, haemoptysis, breathlessness, weight loss, night sweats, malaise, chest pain

3 COPD
cough, sputum, dyspnoea, wheeze

4 Lung tumour
cough, haemoptysis, dyspnoea, chest pain, recurrent or slow resolving pneumonia, anorexia, weight loss

5 Pulmonary embolism
acute breathlessness, pleuritic chest pain, haemoptysis, dizziness, syncope

6 Mesothelioma
chest pain (dull ache, 'boring', diffuse, occasionally pleuritic), dyspnoea, weight loss, profuse sweating, asymptomatic

2 What tests / investigations would you want to do for the condition you have chosen?

3 What treatment would be suitable in each case?

Speaking

1 Work in pairs. Write down a scenario for a patient presenting with the symptoms and signs in *Signs and symptoms* and decide on a cause.

2 Work with a pair who have prepared a different scenario. Swap scenarios and prepare your role as a patient for your new scenario.

3 Take turns taking the history from the patient and explaining the tests in *Signs and symptoms* **2**. Then explain the results and treatment.

4 Work in groups of four. While two doctors do the role-play, one doctor uses a copy of the speaking checklist on page 117 to monitor the doctor and give feedback at the end on agreed criteria. The fourth doctor listens for correct examples of the use of the articles and incorrect use.

5 Two doctors volunteer to do a role-play in front of the class. The class chooses a scenario where a patient thinks he / she has one of the conditions 1–6 in *Signs and symptoms* but the diagnosis is bronchitis or a bad viral flu. The doctor reassures the patient that it is not the condition he / she fears. The role-play may include all or part of the following: the history, the investigations, the diagnosis, or the treatment.

USEFUL EXPRESSIONS
From what you have told me, ...
It looks as if you have ...
If you had ... , you'd ...
Patients with ... usually have ...
It doesn't sound pleasant, but ...
Because your friend had ...
If it doesn't go away, come back and see me.

Reading

1 Work in groups. Before you look at the text, describe Figure 1, which shows the flow–volume loop.

2 Use these words to complete 1–7 in the text.

peak expiratory flow rate   inspiration
closing volume   dynamic compression
fixed upper airway narrowing
expiration   peak flow

3 Work in pairs. Find these phrases in the text. Are they causes or effects?
1 and hence the airways are at their most open
2 the highest flow rates are possible at the beginning of the blow
3 and are less able to resist dynamic compression
4 Also, increasingly with age, the small airways may actually close off
5 the inspiratory muscles are approaching the end of their 'travel'

Flow–volume loop

A good starting point to the understanding of lung function tests is the flow-volume loop. This plots inspiratory and expiratory flow against lung volume during a maximal expiratory and maximal inspiratory manoeuvre. At the beginning of the ¹_____ from a full breath in, the expiratory muscles are at their strongest, the lungs at their biggest, and hence the airways are at their most open. (A). Because the lungs are at their largest, the radial attachments to the airways, effectively the alveolar / capillary membranes and their connective tissue, are pulling the hardest and supporting the airways against ²_____ during the exhalation manoeuvre.

This means that the highest flow rates are possible at the beginning of the blow, hence the sudden rise to a ³_____ in the 100 ms or so of the forced breath out. (B). This is the ⁴_____ and is essentially what a peak flow meter measures.

As the lung empties, and the lung volume drops, the dilatory pull on the airways from the radial attachments of the surrounding lung tissue reduces. (C). Hence the airways narrow and become less supported, and are less able to resist dynamic compression. This means that the maximal airflow obtainable, regardless of effort, falls too.

Eventually, the expiratory muscles come to the end of their 'travel' and cannot squeeze the chest any more. Also, increasingly with age, the small airways may actually close off, preventing any more emptying. (D). The volume at which this begins is called the ⁵_____.

As maximal ⁶_____ starts, although the inspiratory muscles are at their strongest, the airways are at their smallest. Thus, flow rates start low and increase as the airways open up. However, as the airways open up, the inspiratory muscles are approaching the end of their 'travel' and are weakening. This means the flow rates fall again; hence, the different rounded appearance of the inspiratory limb of the flow-volume curve.

Thus, normally the inspiratory and expiratory flow rates depend on lung volume and are termed 'volume-dependent'. If there is ⁷_____, such as from a fibrous tumour in the trachea, then the size of the airway at this point may become so narrow that it now limits maximal flows.

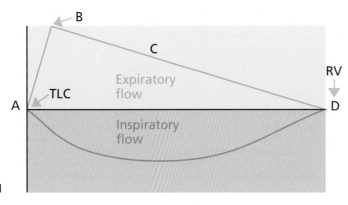

Fig.1

It is now estimated that as many as 300 million people suffer from asthma. British children are three times more likely to suffer asthma than those from France, Germany, or Italy. The highest prevalence rates for asthma in the world are found in the UK, New Zealand, Australia, Ireland, and Canada. Nepal, Romania, Albania, Indonesia, and Macau have the lowest prevalence rates of asthma.
– *GINA (Global Initiative for Asthma)*

Speaking

1 Work in pairs. Describe the device below.

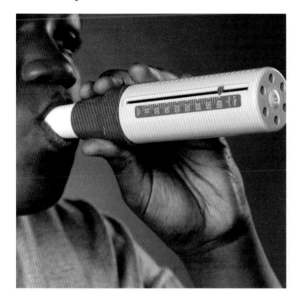

2 Make a list of the steps involved in explaining to a patient how to use a peak flow meter. Take turns explaining to each other using the picture in **1** and these expressions.

USEFUL EXPRESSIONS
You need to …
Can you stand or sit upright?
Ensure the meter is set at …
Take a deep breath.
Seal your lips around it.
Blow out as hard and as fast possible.
Record the best of three efforts.
Repeat.

3 Explain to the patient how to record the readings appropriately using the chart.

PEAK FLOW READINGS CHART

Date and time	Peak flow	% of best	Activity effect	Cough	Wheeze	Short. of breath	Tight chest	Medicine used	Notes
Mon, 01 Aug 2005 12:00 PM	503	87%				XX			
Sun, 31 Jul 2005 12:00 PM	480	83%	X	X	X	X			
Sat, 30 Jul 2005 12:00 PM	541	94%							
Fri, 29 Jul 2005 12:00 PM	516	89%		X		X			
Thu, 28 Jul 2005 12:00 PM	483	84%		X	X	X			
Wed, 27 Jul 2005 12:00 PM	565	98%			X	XX			
Tue, 26 Jul 2005 12:00 PM	497	86%		X	X	X			
Mon, 25 Jul 2005 12:00 PM	273	47%	XXX	X	XXX	XX	X	XXX	
Sun, 24 Jul 2005 12:00 PM	501	87%	X	X					
Sat, 23 Jul 2005 12:00 PM	540	93%	X	X	X	X			
Fri, 22 Jul 2005 12:00 PM	537	93%	X	X	X				
Thu, 21 Jul 2005 12:00 PM	471	81%	X			X			
Wed, 20 Jul 2005 12:00 PM	547	95%							
Tue, 19 Jul 2005 12:00 PM	544	94%	X	X					
Mon, 18 Jul 2005 12:00 PM	470	81%							
Sun, 17 Jul 2005 12:00 PM	500	86%		X		XX			
Sat, 16 Jul 2005 12:00 PM	480	83%	X	X	X	X			
Fri, 15 Jul 2005 12:00 PM	475	82%		X	X	X			
Thu, 14 Jul 2005 12:00 PM	520	90%				X			
Wed, 13 Jul 2005 12:00 PM	370	64%	X	X	X	XX	X	XXX	
Tue, 12 Jul 2005 12:00 PM	496	86%	X	X	X				
Mon, 11 Jul 2005 12:00 PM	562	97%							

X = Mild or occasional symptoms   XX = Medium or frequent symptoms   XXX = Severe or continuous symptoms

Project

1 Work in pairs. Find information on the internet on explaining the use of inhalers to patients. Or choose one of the sites below.
- www.patient.co.uk
- Asthma UK: www.asthma.org.uk
- American Society of Chest Physicians: www.chestnet.org
- British Thoracic Society: www.brit-thoracic.org.uk
- European Respiratory Society: www.ersnet.org
- Society of Thoracic Surgeons: www.sts.org
- BTS training site: www.chestnet.net
- For simple thoracic anatomy and other anatomy see: anatomy.uams.edu

Also check the *Oxford Handbook of Clinical Examination and Practical Skills.*

2 Share and compare the information with other students and choose the best resource.

Listening 3

Explaining a device

1 🎧 Listen to a nurse explaining to a patient how to use a breath-activated pressurized MDI (Metered Dose Inhaler). Write down the verbs the nurse uses to explain how to use the device after she says: *First of all, you remove the cap …*

2 Work in pairs. Compare lists and check with other students to complete your list.

3 🎧 The nurse asks the patient to explain the procedure to her. The following illustrations show what the patient explained to the nurse. Listen again to the nurse's explanation. Which three steps are not illustrated?

4 Work in pairs. Compare answers.

Speaking

Work in pairs. Take turns explaining to the patient how to use the breath-activated inhaler and then ask the patient to explain it to you. The patient should make some mistakes. Correct the patient politely.

USEFUL EXPRESSIONS
OK, that's fine, but try to do it like this.
Do you want to show me again?
Fine, just try doing it like this.
OK, just see if you can do it like this.
That's nearly it.
Can you try it again for me?

Writing

Describing data

1 Work by yourself. Look at the chart opposite which shows trends in annual rates of primary care consultations, hospital admissions, and mortality for asthma among children under five. Which line or lines on the chart do these words and phrases relate to?

1 trends overall
2 experience a steady decline almost to zero
3 increase substantially during
4 halve
5 more than halve
6 reach a high, throughout the period
7 hospital admission rate
8 rise sharply
9 upward trend
10 downward trend overall with the exception of

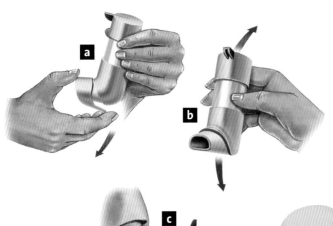

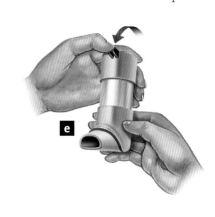

Key words

Adjectives
barking
breath-activated
expiratory
hoarse
hollow
inspiratory
offensive
productive
purulent
tenacious
tickly

Nouns
bronchitis
crackles
expectoration
high
malaise
MDI
sputum
trend

Useful reference

Oxford Handbook of Respiratory Medicine
2nd edition, Chapman et al,
ISBN 978-019-954516-2

Asthma and allergies: decrease in hospital admissions in 1990s

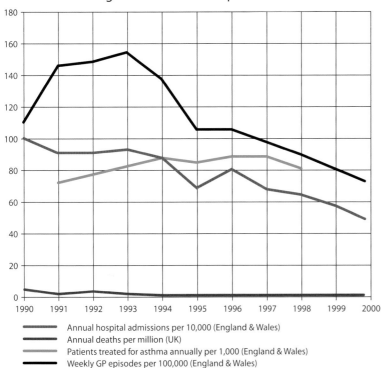

Annual hospital admissions per 10,000 (England & Wales)
Annual deaths per million (UK)
Patients treated for asthma annually per 1,000 (England & Wales)
Weekly GP episodes per 100,000 (England & Wales)

Trends in annual rates of primary care consultations, hospital admissions, and mortality for asthma among children aged under fiver years

2 Work in groups. Check your answers. Together prepare orally a description of the data of between 150 and 200 words, using the phrases below. At this stage do not write, but you may make notes.

USEFUL EXPRESSIONS
The graph / chart shows / illustrates / provides information about / provides a breakdown of ...
Generally speaking, the trends ..., with the exception of ...,
For example, / For instance,... / Take ..., for example.
Similarly, / Likewise, / Furthermore ,...
As regards / Regarding / With regard to / As can be seen / Turning to ...
By contrast / Compared to / In comparison with / By comparison
Respectively
As against / As opposed to

3 On your own, write a description of the data using the simple past. Quote the data to support your description. You do not need to describe every change in the chart.

11 Tropical diseases

Check up

1 Describe these pictures. What relevance do they have for the spread of infectious diseases?

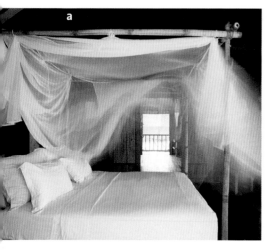

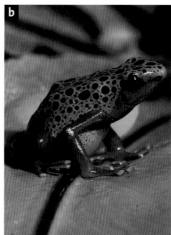

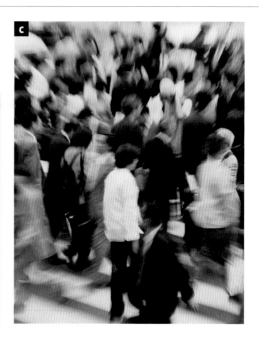

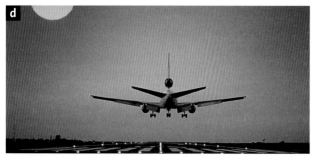

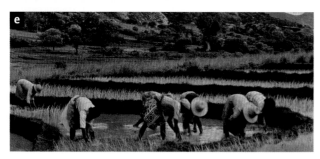

2 Work in groups. In the UK certain diseases are notifiable. What types of diseases do you think have to be notified to the authorities and why do they have to be notified? Do you have the same system in your country?

3 What epidemics / pandemics do you know in the world since the beginning of the twentieth century?

Project

1 Work in groups. Use your own knowledge and the internet to find out more information about these milestones in public health practice nationally and internationally.

1 1600s – Variolation (the induction of mild smallpox to reduce mortality, an ancient practice in Asia) spreads to Africa, Europe, the Ottoman Empire, and the Americas.

2 1796 – Edward Jenner immunizes James Phipps with cowpox virus.

3 1854 – John Snow shows that cholera spreads through contaminated drinking water.

4 1873 – Henrik Arnhauer Hansen identifies the bacillus causing leprosy under microscope.

5 1882 – Koch discovers the bacillus causing tuberculosis.

6 1887 – Ronald Ross in India describes the malaria–mosquito life cycle.

7 1928 – Fleming discovers the antibacterial effect of penicillin.

8 1953 – Polio vaccine introduced.

2 Share the information you have found with the class.

Speaking

1 Work in pairs. Choose the three most important developments in *Project* 1. Rank them in order of importance.

2 Compare your rankings with other pairs. Are their rankings similar to yours?

3 Choose the most important development from the list.

USEFUL EXPRESSIONS
If it were not for ...   If ... hadn't ...,
... is the single most ...   By far, the most ...

Listening 1

Treating returning travellers

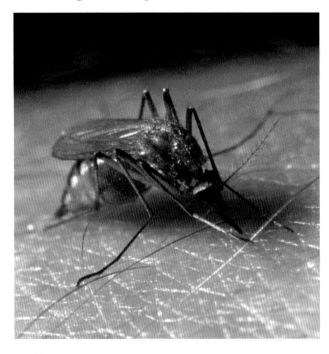

1 🎧 Listen to the talk on treating illness among returning travellers. Look at the notes and the picture above and decide what the illness is.

2 Work in pairs. Look at the notes made by a student. What is the part of speech (noun, verb, etc.) of each of the missing words?

3 What do the abbreviations stand for? Use a dictionary or ask a partner.

4 🎧 Listen again and complete the notes made by a student during the presentation. In each space write no more than three words from the talk.

With travellers coming back from holidays important to think about ¹_____

In history, need to ask about
- the symptoms
- areas travelled to (including brief stopovers)
- the duration of the travel
- immunizations received ²_____
- malaria prophylaxis
- health of members of the ³_____
- sexual contacts whilst abroad
- medical treatment received abroad.

Full examination should be given.

Investigations, think about FBC, thick and thin ⁴_____ for malaria, LFTs, viral serology, blood culture, stool culture (ensure it is fresh), MSU.

Malaria

⁵_____ are notified each year in the UK

Easy to miss diagnosis

Great ⁶_____ – can present with nearly any symptoms

⁷_____ of headache, malaise, myalgia, and anorexia, followed by recurring fevers, rigors, and ⁸_____, which last for 8–12 hours at a time

5 What questions would you ask in taking the history of a businessman who had been to South America and presented with fever?

6 Work in pairs and take turns taking the history from each other.

The Health Protection Agency has a useful A–Z of topics at www.hpa.org.uk

Vocabulary

Travellers' diarrhoea

1 Complete the text using these adjectives.

chlorinated   contaminated   frequent
hyper-osmolar   preferable   reputable
self-limiting   sweetened   unhygienic
unpeeled

Management
- Most episodes are [1]_____.
- Increase fluid intake. Eating e.g. broth with noodles or salty crackers with [2]_____ drinks will provide a balance of carbohydrate and salt.
- Oral rehydration solution (ORS) is [3]_____ if the diarrhoea is frequent or severe or if there are signs of dehydration, weakness, or muscle cramps.
- Drinks designed for rehydration during sports activities do not contain the correct balance of salts for diarrhoea treatment. Sodas and fruit juices are often [4]_____ or have high sugar content and can make diarrhoea worse.
- Prompt antibiotic treatment reduces symptom duration.
- Loperamide shortens the episode in older children and adults with [5]_____ small volume stools. (Do not use loperamide if there is blood in the stools, fever, tenesmus, or other signs of dysentery.)

Prevention
Avoid [6]_____ fruit, uncooked vegetables, sauces which are not freshly prepared and handled in [7]_____ conditions e.g. by street vendors. Where there is no reliable source of [8]_____ water, sterilize water by boiling or with chlorine tablets or drink bottled water from a [9]_____ source. Avoid bottled water where the bottles are immersed in water or ice to keep them cool. Beware ice or ice cream, which may be made using [10]_____ water. When trekking or in isolated places, it is advisable to carry packets of ORS and a course of treatment. Hand sanitizers are useful when hand-washing is impossible.

2 Work in pairs. Take turns explaining to another doctor the management or prevention of travellers' diarrhoea. Then explain the management or prevention to a patient.

Speaking

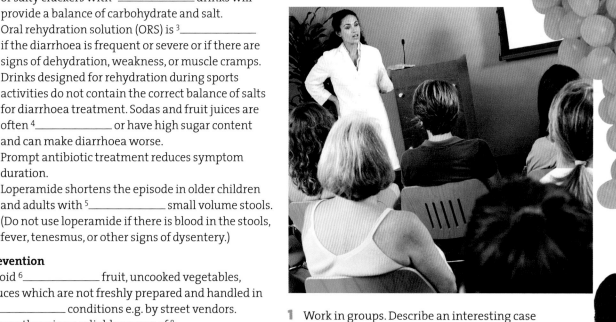

1 Work in groups. Describe an interesting case presentation of a patient who had a disease that is not prevalent in Western Europe or one that is not prevalent in your country. Say what you learnt from the case and what you would do differently if you had to do it again.

2 Choose one student from each group to describe their case to the rest of the class. If possible, use PowerPoint or the electronic smartboard.

3 Work on your own. Write a description of no more than 150–200 words of the case you described. Describe the sequence of events and add what you learnt from it and how you would improve your performance if you did it again.

Remember always to maintain patient confidentiality.

● **Language spot**
Linking words

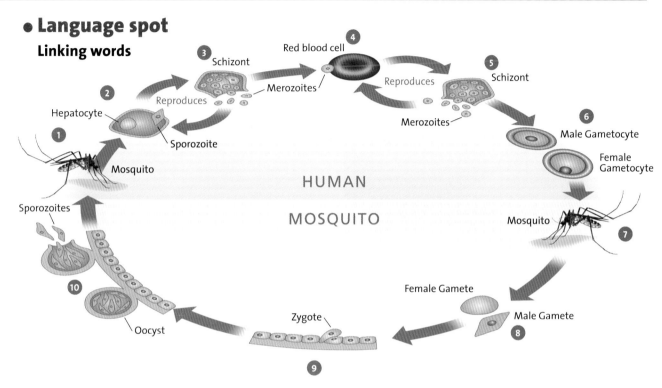

1 Work in pairs. Look at the diagram of the life cycle of the malarial parasite. Describe steps 1–5 in your own words.

2 Read this description of the same steps. Underline the words that are suitable in each case. In some cases more than one is suitable.

> The sexual part of the life cycle of the malarial mosquito takes place in the invertebrate host (the Anopheles mosquito) and the asexual cycle occurs in the vertebrate host (the human).
> At the vertebrate stage, [1]*when / where / then* the mosquito needs blood for her eggs, she bites the human host and at the same time injects motile sporozoites into the blood stream. [2]*After that / Next / Then* these invade hepatocytes, [3]*where / when / then* they develop into liver schizonts. [4]*When / As soon as / Next* each schizont ruptures, thousands of merozoites are released. [5]*After that / Once / After this* happens, the merozoites invade red blood cells. This [6] *after that / next / then* triggers the part of the cycle which is responsible for all the clinical manifestations of the disease.

3 Work in pairs and describe steps 6–10.

➤➤ Go to **Grammar reference** p 126

Writing
Describing a life cycle

1 Work in pairs. Write about 150 words describing steps 6–10 in the life cycle of the malarial parasite in the diagram in *Language spot*.

2 Compare your answer with another pair of students. Check each other's writing for mistakes.

USEFUL WORDS AND EXPRESSIONS
At the next step / stage / phase ...
Following that ...
Afterwards ...
Before ...

deoxygenated (adj) having oxygen removed

infarct (n) an area of cell death / necrosis which is caused by an obstruction of the local blood supply. Another word for *infarction*.

dactylitis (n) inflammation of the fingers and toes

Reading

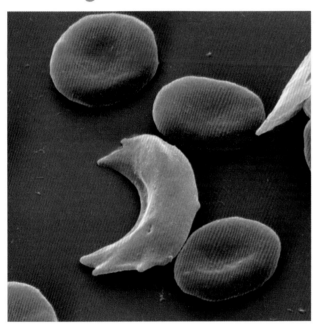

1 Work in groups. Before you look at the text, look at the titles and pool your knowledge on sickle-cell anaemia. Predict what you expect to see in the reading passage.

2 Find words in the passage which mean:
  1 to break down or disintegrate
  2 combine with another compound to form a polymer
  3 characteristic
  4 interchange
  5 blocking
  6 accompanying or occurring with
  7 brought on
  8 develops later
  9 change.

Sickle-cell anaemia

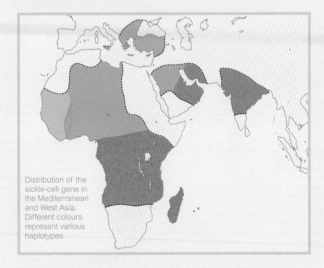

Distribution of the sickle-cell gene in the Mediterranean and West Asia. Different colours represent various haplotypes.

The sickle-cell gene is common in equatorial Africa (frequency 25%), Saudi Arabia, and south Asia but less common in the Mediterranean and the mixed populations of the Americas (frequency 5%). It is due to a single point mutation in the Hb β-globin gene chain. When deoxygenated, HbS molecules polymerize into elongated structures causing erythrocytes to deform and haemolyze. Sickled red cells are rigid and block the micro-circulation in various organs, causing infarcts.

The inheritance of the disease is autosomal co-dominant (i.e. sickle-cell disease is due to heterozygous inheritance HbAS). The trait is generally asymptomatic. Sickle-cell disease occurs with homozygous inheritance of the gene (HbSS) or co-inheritance of another β-globin chain disorder such as HbC (see below). Sickle-cell disease and glucose–phosphate dehydrogenase (G6PD) deficiency may occur together because of the high prevalence of both conditions in some regions. They provide protection against malaria.

Clinical features of sickle-cell anaemia

Severe haemolytic anaemia is punctuated by severe pain crises. Young patients alternate periods of good health with acute crises. Later chronic ill health supervenes due to organ damage. Symptoms begin after six months of age as the HbF level declines. The first signs are often of acute dactylitis due to occlusive necrosis of the small bones of the hands and feet, resulting in digits of varying length. The long bones are affected in older children and adults. Anaemia (Hb 6-8 g/dl; reticulocytes 10-20%) is well tolerated because of cardiac compensation and a lower affinity of HbS for oxygen.

CNS central nervous system
CXR chest X-ray

The severity of complications depends on a number of factors including the proportion of non-sickle Hb molecules (e.g. HbF) and the ratio α to β chains, which may be modified by concomitant α thalassaemia trait or conditions affecting β-globin chain production (Bantu haplotype is associated with severe disease, whilst Senegalese and Asian haplotypes are less severe).

Types of crises

● Painful vascular-occlusive: frequent and precipitated by infections, acidosis, dehydration, or hypoxia. Infarcts often occur in the axial skeleton, lungs, and spleen. Repeated splenic infarction leads to hyposplenism in adulthood. Crises can involve the CNS (in 7% of the patients) and spinal cord.

● Visceral sequestration: due to sickling within organs and pooling of blood.

● Chest: pulmonary infiltrates on CXR, fever, chest pain, tachypnoea, cough, wheeze. There is often concomitant infection, microvascular occlusion, and bronchoconstriction. Chest crises can arise during a painful crisis; patients should be monitored carefully for this complication, which can be fatal.

● Haemolytic: raised rate of haemolysis with a fall in Hb. Usually accompanying a painful crisis. Concomitant G6PD deficiency may worsen haemolysis.

● Aplastic: Arrest of red cell production due to infection with parvovirus and / or folate deficiency. It is characterized by a sudden fall in Hb and reticulocytes, emergency blood transfusion can be life-saving.

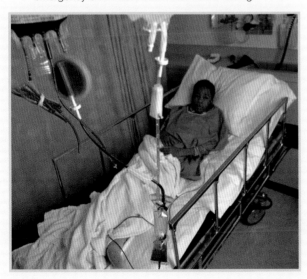

3 Work in pairs. Are the statements true or false?

1 The sickle-cell gene is as widespread in the Americas as it is in Africa.
2 Infarcts can be caused when sickled red cells obstruct circulation in certain organs.
3 Sickle-cell disease and G6PD combined protect sufferers against malaria.
4 The first signs of severe haemolytic anaemia are always seen in the bones and hands of the feet.
5 The severity of the complications is linked to the proportion of non-sickle Hb molecules.
6 Patients can die when a chest crisis occurs during a painful crisis.
7 During an aplastic crisis, a blood transfusion always saves lives.

4 Work in groups. How common is sickle-cell anaemia in your country? Have you treated cases of this condition? Give examples.

Listening 2
Maintaining good health

1 🎧 Listen to the conversation between Dr Lindt and Mrs Boyce. What is the subject of the conversation?

2 🎧 Listen again. Write down as many details as you can.

3 🎧 Work in pairs. Compare your answers with a colleague and if necessary listen again.

4 Work in groups. Describe the best ways for patients with sickle-cell disease to maintain good health. Make notes and share your information with the class.

5 Work in pairs. You are a GP and you are going to talk to a patient, Mr(s) Dillon, about the best ways to maintain good health for himself / herself. Using the notes from 2 and 4 above, take turns role-playing the conversation.

USEFUL EXPRESSIONS
It's important ...   You need to ...
Where possible try to ...   If you (do this) ..., then ...
If you get (sick, especially high fever) ..., contact ...
immediately. Don't wait.

Physiotherapy should never be painful. The expression 'No pain, no gain' has no place in physiotherapy.
– *Oxford Handbook of Tropical Medicine*

Stroke

One of the complications of sickle-cell anaemia is stroke. Rehabilitation and physiotherapy after stroke is essential 24 hours a day and as the physiotherapy can be undone by bad posture during the night and at other times, it is a good idea to teach the relatives the basics of physiotherapy.

Patient care

1 Work in pairs. Look at the diagrams, which show positioning and movements for hemiplegic patients lying down. Decide what instructions you would give to someone to explain how to position a hemiplegic relative.

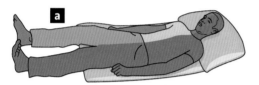

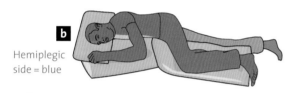

Hemiplegic side = blue

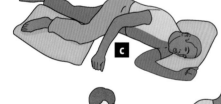

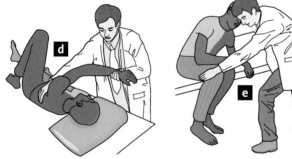

2 Match these sentences to the pictures in 1.

1 Help Andrew to get up to sit on the bed.
2 Position Andrew on the stroke (hemiplegic) side like this with a cushion under the head and leg like this.
3 Roll Andrew onto his normal side while supporting his weak shoulder.
4 Lay Andrew on the normal side like this with cushions under the stroke (hemiplegic) arm and leg.
5 Position and cushion Andrew in the supine position.

3 Work in pairs. Take turns explaining to a relative how to position and support a patient who has suffered a stroke. Use the diagrams above to help you.

Speaking

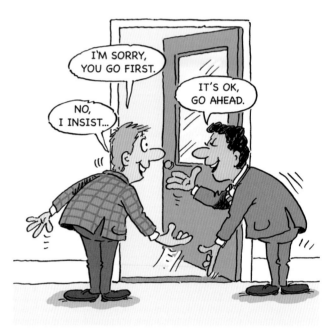

1 Work in groups. Look at statements 1–10 and match them with a–g.

1 Do you want to add anything to that?
2 Ahmed, what about you?
3 I agree with what you said but, what about ... ?
4 Can I just say that ... ?
5 I think you're right, but we also need to think about ...
6 I think that's it exactly.
7 I'm not so sure if that's going to work.
8 Any more suggestions or ideas from anyone?
9 No, I'm sorry. It's OK. You go first.
10 Shall we appoint someone to take notes?

a agreeing
b disagreeing
c agreeing and disagreeing
d inviting someone to speak
e adding information
f apologizing for speaking over someone
g taking the lead in the discussion

2 Can you add any more expressions of your own to the list above?

3 Look at the task below, which is an awareness exercise for GPs working in areas with patients from a wide range of backgrounds. Spend several minutes thinking about the task. Make mental notes about the measures, but don't write anything down.

> You are working in a general practice in the UK which covers an area where there are many patients who have come from or whose families have come from South America, Africa, and south-east Asia. You do not feel that the GP practice is catering well for these patients. What are the three best measures to improve the situation?

4 Work in groups of three or four. Each group should pair with another group, one as group A and the other as group B. Group A discusses the task in **3** and decides on the three best solutions. Each student in Group B monitors the performance of a student in group A. After fifteen minutes of discussion, the students each give feedback in pairs on the performance using the following criteria: *ability at turn taking, respect for colleagues, contribution to the discussion, teamwork.*

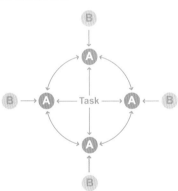

5 Change roles and this time the students in group B discuss while those in A monitor.

6 Choose the best measure to improve the situation.

12 Technology

Check up

1 Describe these pictures.

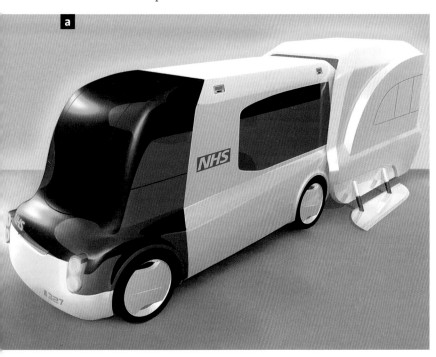

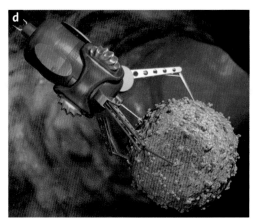

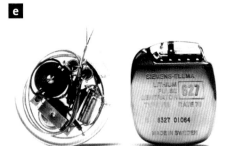

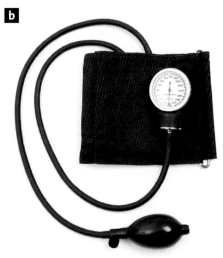

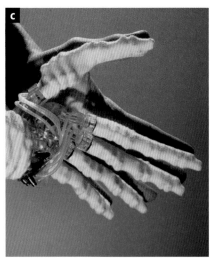

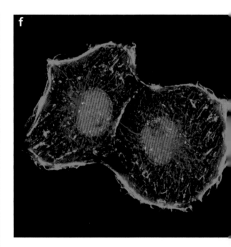

2 Work in groups. What are the main advantages and disadvantages of technology?

3 Some people think that deskilling and losing sight of the patient are the main downsides of the use of technology in medicine. Do you agree?

4 Why do people often resist the introduction of new technology? Give examples from your own experience. What are the reactions to innovations in science and medicine in particular in your country?

Vocabulary

Change

1 Work in pairs. Which two adjectives in italics can you use together to complete each sentence? Are the two adjectives you chose in the correct order?

1 Technology like computers has brought about *structural / big / far-reaching* **change** in the provision of health care internationally.

2 The first face transplant represented a *diplomatic / medical / real* **breakthrough**.

3 In recent years, some very *dramatic / enormous / technological* **advances** have been made in medicine.

4 Throughout history, many *important / recent / medical* **developments** have been curtailed out of fear and ignorance.

5 Keyhole surgery was a(n) *ingenious / modern / latest* **invention**.

6 Society at large, not just the medical field, is undergoing a *computing / complete / technological* **revolution**.

7 A *radical / whole / sudden* **transformation** occurred in the way patients were treated.

8 Stifling *constant / scientific / important* **innovations** in medicine through lack of funding is indefensible.

9 I'd like to find something tracing the *constant / biological / technological* **evolution** of medical science.

10 The government sponsored a *pioneering / latest / joint* **initiative** between the medical schools.

2 Work in pairs. What are the verb forms of the nouns in **bold** in **1**?

Listening 1

Technological advances

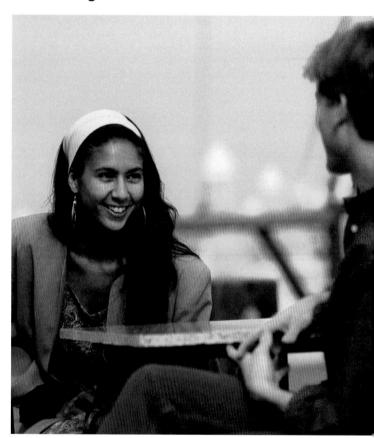

1 🎧 Work in groups. Listen to two doctors, a male and female, discussing technological advances in medicine. Two students (Students A) concentrate on what the female doctor says and two students (Students B) concentrate on the male doctor. Make notes as you listen.

2 Students A, check your notes with each other. Students B, do the same. Then combine your information.

3 🎧 Then listen again and check you have understood everything.

4 Make a list of developments you would like to see in medicine. Describe and evaluate your predictions for the future. Give reasons for your comments.

xeno-transplant (n) animal to human transplant

Vocabulary

Evaluating change

1 Work in groups. Look at the adjectives on page 107 in *Vocabulary* **1**. Which adjectives evaluate the nouns? Which describe?

2 Work out which adjectives are being described below. The words are jumbled upside down below.

1 a synonym of the word dangerous ___z_____
2 to do with being advantageous ___n_____l
3 a synonym for convincing p_____e
4 to do with causing harm _____f___
5 to do with having great worth ___v_____e
6 to do with being easy to use at any time c_____t
7 a synonym for frightening a_____m__
8 to do with not being able to support something i___e_____
9 a synonym for damaging d_____l
10 to do with distasteful o__j_____e

persuasive
objectionable   invaluable   indefensible
hazardous   harmful   detrimental
convenient   beneficial   alarming

3 Which of these words are synonyms of the words in **2**? One word may be used twice.

compelling	helpful	incalculable
offensive	practical	risky
shocking	unjustifiable	unsafe

Speaking

1 Work in groups of four. Discuss which of these issues you think are controversial or sensitive matters for you and for the general public.

- Animal experiments / vivisection
- Xeno-transplants
- Face transplants
- Genetic manipulation
- Growing spare body parts

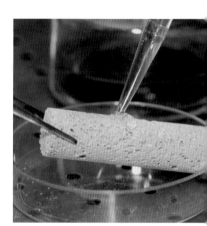

2 Choose a topic from **1** and divide into two sides, for and against. Prepare at least three arguments for each side. Then debate the issue. Discuss also whether the procedure is acceptable in your own country.

USEFUL EXPRESSIONS
arouse emotion / controversy / debate
controversial / sensitive / debatable issue
outweigh / offset / be more important than any /
compensate for

3 Choose a member from one group to summarize both sides of the argument for the rest of the class. Other group members should lend support.

Listening 2

Trying to persuade the doctor

1 🎧 Listen to the five short conversations between a doctor and a patient. Write down the patient's first question in each conversation.

2 Work in pairs. Compare your answers.

3 Work in pairs. Discuss why you think the patients asked the questions that they did. Then check your answers in the *Grammar reference* on page 126.

4 🎧 Listen again. Write down the doctor's reply.

5 Take turns asking each other questions and replying.

Why innovate? Within three years of introduction of the first antiretroviral treatments, AIDS deaths dropped by 70%. Improvements in treatment have helped cut cancer death rates in half.

Vaccines have saved countless children from diseases such as polio, rubella, measles, and tetanus.

– Council for American Medical Innovation

● Language spot

Negative questions

1 Look at the faces. What feelings do you think they are showing?

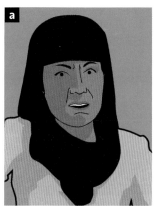
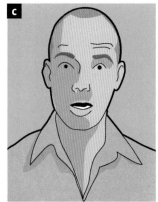
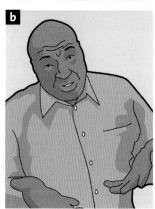
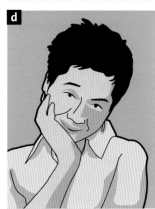

2 Work in pairs. Look at these statements made by patients. What feelings or thoughts could lie behind the questions?

1 Couldn't I just keep using the same device?
2 Isn't this available on the NHS?
3 Wouldn't it be better for me just to continue with medication?
4 Doesn't this device come with a cap on it?
5 Shouldn't my daughter be next?
6 Won't I be having the operation today either?
7 Can't I have an MRI scan?
8 Hasn't the doctor arrived yet?
9 Haven't you done that referral letter yet?
10 Didn't you say I could go home today?
11 Aren't I next on the waiting list?

3 Work in pairs. Match the meanings a–k to the statements 1–11 in **2**.

a You should have.
b He's late.
c I don't like this new one.
d I can't afford to pay for it.
e It's missing.
f I want one.
g I feel angry because it's been cancelled.
h I think you've left me off the waiting list.
i You've kept us waiting too long.
j I don't want to stop.
k I think you've forgotten.

4 🎧 All of the statements in **2** are made by a patient. Work in pairs. Listen and decide which you would put into the categories below. Some may fit into more than one category.

a a strong criticism
b a mild criticism
c a reminder
d avoiding criticism
e showing shock / surprise
f persuasion / a demand

5 Decide how you would reply to each statement in **2**.

USEFUL EXPRESSIONS
You could / can, but …
I'm afraid not, because …
Oh, yes, sorry …
Oh, yes, you're right.
I'm very sorry, but …
Yes, we have.
I did, but …

6 Work in pairs. Take turns asking and replying to the questions. Develop the answers in your own way.

7 Can you think of acceptable and unacceptable examples of situations where you can use negative questions like those in **2** with colleagues? Give reasons. Look at the audio script for *Listening* 2 on page 137.

>> Go to **Grammar reference** p 126

Speaking

1 Work in pairs. Look at the photos. You have two patients. One patient is insisting on having each of the procedures or items in the photos and the other is reluctant to have them. Decide what the patient might say in each case.

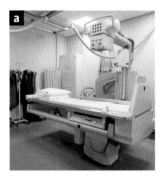

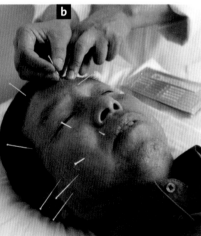

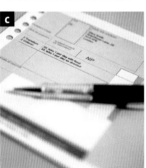

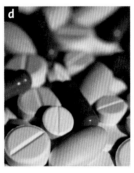

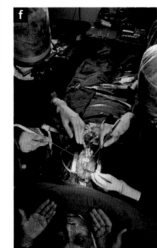

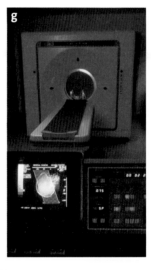

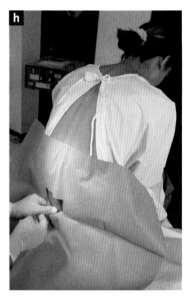

2 Work in pairs. Take turns role-playing the conversation between the doctor and the patient. The patient can be difficult and insistent.

Reading

1 Work in pairs. Look at the three extracts on page 111. What do you think is the source of each text?

2 Match these sources to the extracts 1–3.

A newspaper
A website for patients
A specialist website on stem cell research

3 Replace the highlighted words in these sentences with a word from the extracts.

1 Scientists learnt how to grow stem cells in the laboratory after years of experimentation.

2 Stem cell treatment involves hazards as well as being harsh.

3 Professor Dhillon's reaction is unambiguous when asked if the research at Edinburgh met any resistance.

4 As it is connected with the use of foetuses, the term *stem cell* is quite sensitive to many people.

5 Patients are given information as to when the advantages are greater than the dangers in a stem cell transplant.

harvest (v) (of tissue or organs) collect
unspecialized (adj) of cells, not differentiated

Do not go where the path may lead, go instead
where there is no path and leave a trail.
– *Ralph Waldo Emerson, 1803–1882*

Extract 1

Stem Cell Transplant

A stem cell transplant is used to increase the chance of a cure or remission for a number of cancers and blood disorders. It usually involves intense chemotherapy followed by an infusion of stem cells. The treatment requires close nursing and medical care for a number of weeks. It can be a gruelling treatment and there are risks. Your specialist can advise when the likely benefits of this procedure can outweigh the risks.

What is a stem cell transplant?

A stem cell transplant may be used so that you can have intensive high dose chemotherapy (and sometimes radiotherapy) to kill cancerous cells. The chemotherapy is higher than conventional chemotherapy and also kills the stem cells in the bone marrow that would normally make blood cells. Therefore, following the chemotherapy, you are given back (transplanted) stem cells which can then make normal blood cells again.

A stem cell transplant is sometimes called a bone marrow transplant. However, stem cells can be obtained from blood as well as from the bone marrow. So, the term *stem cell transplant* is now used.

Extract 2

Stem cell research is a subject almost guaranteed to prompt mixed reactions. As if to illustrate that fact, two high-profile Scottish stem cell trials were announced this week, to very different responses. While one was branded 'immoral and unethical' by critics, the other was warmly welcomed as offering a potential cure for some types of blindness.

The difference is that the former – a trial in Glasgow to insert stem cells into the brains of stroke victims – relies on stem cells harvested from human embryos, which must be destroyed to enable the beginning of a cell line.

Edinburgh uses stem cells from voluntary adult donors, harvested after their death, to treat corneal blindness. It is the use of voluntary adult donors that makes all the difference to those with moral and ethical objections to stem cell therapy.

Asked if he had encountered any opposition, Prof Dhillon is unequivocal. 'No. Because we're using tissue that's been generously donated by adult donors after death, those issues don't arise with this type of research.

'I think the term *stem cell* has become rather emotive in that it's linked with a number of images and issues, both ethical and moral, associated with the use of foetuses, and this trial is not using foetal stem cells. But I think it's important for clinicians, scientists, and the public to have an open debate.'

Extract 3

The specific factors and conditions that allow stem cells to remain unspecialized are of great interest to scientists. It has taken scientists many years of trial and error to learn to grow stem cells in the laboratory without them spontaneously differentiating into specific cell types. For example, it took twenty years to learn how to grow human embryonic stem cells in the laboratory following the development of conditions for growing mouse stem cells. Therefore an important area of research is understanding the signals in a mature organism that cause a stem cell population to proliferate and remain unspecialized until the cells are needed for repair of a specific tissue. Such information is critical for scientists to be able to grow large numbers of unspecialized stem cells in the laboratory for further experimentation.

4 Answer these questions.

1 Why is it important for scientists to understand the signals in a mature organism that cause a stem cell population to proliferate and remain unspecialized until the cells are needed for repair of a specific tissue?

2 Why has the Edinburgh trial not had a negative response to its work?

3 What difference is mentioned between normal chemotherapy and that used in stem cell transplants?

5 Work in groups. Are you interested in genetics? Give reasons and examples.

demystify (v) take away the mystery about something; to make something clear

Pandora's box (n) a process that, if started, will cause many problems that cannot be solved

Frankenstein (n) a fictional doctor who assembled a human from the parts of dead people, resulting in a creature often called 'Frankentein's Monster'

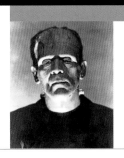

The novel *Frankenstein*, published in 1818, was written by Mary Shelley.

Speaking

1 Work in pairs. Look at the picture and describe what is happening.

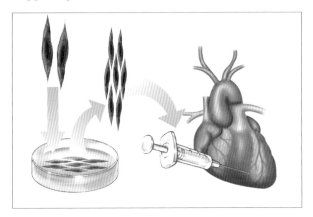

2 Work in pairs. Is each statement for or against stem cell therapies?

1 Stem cell research is the breakthrough that sufferers of illnesses and paralysis have been waiting for.

2 The best way to approach the issue is to clarify how the procedure works to make people feel at ease with stem cell research. Once it has been demystified, people are more likely to accept it.

3 Stem cell research and therapies are indefensible because they interfere with nature.

4 Many people are apprehensive about harvesting stem cells from embryos to use in any kind of treatment.

5 I can understand the faith people have in stem cell therapy, but I think it is a step too far both ethically and scientifically.

6 Provided there are sufficient safeguards in place, stem cell research is surely a welcome development.

7 A development like stem cell research is scientifically complex and has such dangerous consequences that it's impossible to allay people's fears.

8 Stem cell research and therapy give hope to thousands of sufferers.

3 Decide which category of statements you agree with. Then compare your answers with another pair of students.

4 Discuss the main arguments for and against stem cell research / therapy from the ethical and scientific view. Look at the words and ideas below.

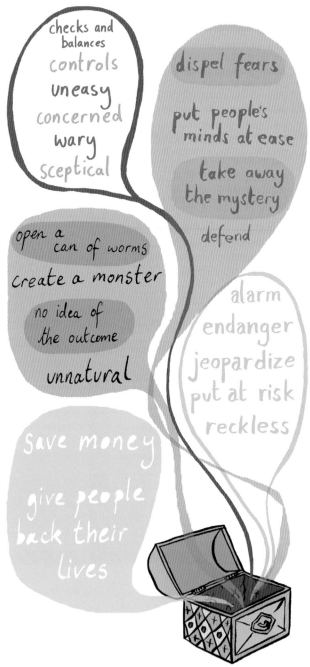

checks and balances
controls
uneasy
concerned
wary
sceptical

dispel fears
put people's minds at ease
take away the mystery
defend

open a can of worms
create a monster
no idea of the outcome
unnatural

alarm
endanger
jeopardize
put at risk
reckless

save money
give people back their lives

5 Make a master list of ideas in **4** for the whole class.

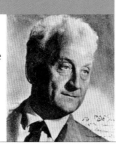

Discovery consists of seeing what everybody else has seen and thinking what nobody else has thought.
– *Albert von Szent-Györgyi 1893–1986, Hungarian biochemist*

Writing

Stem cell therapy

1 Work in pairs. Look at the text on stem cell therapy. Complete the text by inserting these phrases.

a these innovations
b not just objectionable, but dangerous
c a major breakthrough in medical science
d the knock-on effect
e and other important medical advances

Stem cell therapy is ¹_____ which offers new hope for stroke victims as well as for sufferers of many other conditions. However, the benefits are not just limited to the patient, but extend to the carer, often a family member, and the health care system. From the family's point of view the patient would be given their lives back and would possibly even be able to lead an active life and work again. For the carer, there is the release from the burden of care and the possibility of finding work.

The cost of medical care will be brought down with a reduction in community support, the supply of medications and equipment like hoists, and home modifications. The time spent in hospital will also be reduced. So in a short time the research will soon pay for itself. Then there is ²_____ of being able to use the money saved to pay for other areas of treatment. It must be emphasized that the health care system will only gain from ³_____ if any changes are well managed and the benefits spread around.

Some people, however, have reservations about this ⁴_____ that have taken place in recent years, primarily from the ethical point of view. They feel that stem cell research is ⁵_____.

2 Work on your own and continue the third paragraph. Compare your answer with a partner.

Checklist

Assess your progress in this unit.
Tick (✓) the statements which are true.

I can understand and use vocabulary about change

I can evaluate change and development

I can ask and deal with negative questions

I can write about arguments

Key words

Adjectives
alarming
beneficial
compelling
emotive
far-reaching
hazardous
ingenious
objectionable
persuasive
radical
reckless
sensitive
uneasy
unequivocal
unjustifiable

Nouns
breakthrough
criticism
development
revolution

Useful reference

Oxford Handbook of Clinical Medicine, 7th edition, Longmore et al, ISBN 978-0-19-856837-7

Speaking activities

Student A

Unit 1 p.7

You are the brother / sister of a 22-year-old male / female whom you witnessed passing out in a shop. This is the first time it happened. Your brother / sister had no prodrome; a cry followed by tonic / clonic movements; post-ictal drowsiness, confusion, cyanosis, frothing from the mouth, incontinence, aching limbs; slow recovery lasting about twenty minutes.

Add any further information from your own medical knowledge.

Possible diagnosis: epilepsy, but need to rule out other possibilities.

Unit 3 p.23

Your notes

30 years of age male / female, pain in the elbow, left-handed, goes to the gym, plays / squash and some weights, has RSI when at work, pains in the wrist, doesn't use support, tennis, not go to the gym, play in the park, flare up joints

Unit 5 p.42

You are Mrs Buxton. You gave birth to a baby ten days ago. You present to the GP's surgery with a little bit of tearfulness which has gone on longer than the first few days after giving birth, but is nothing serious. You are getting a lot of support from your friends and family. You
- laugh at things as per normal
- look forward to things
- know things not your fault even if get on top of you
- are sometimes anxious / worried but normal
- are sometimes panicky, but no more than normal
- are coping quite well
- have no problem sleeping
- are not sad a lot
- cried a little first few days, then perked up, then started again; not a lot, but it's there
- have never thought of harming yourself.

Unit 7 p.69

Choose one of the pictures and show it to the doctor at the appropriate moment.

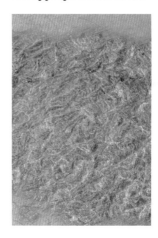
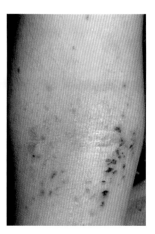

Unit 9 p.85

You are a 45-year-old patient who has pericarditis. You are anxious and have the following:

Sharp chest pain, central retrosternal, worse on deep inspiration, change in position, exercise and swallowing, pericardial effusion may cause dysphagia by pressing the oesophagus.

At the appropriate point show the doctor the ECG.

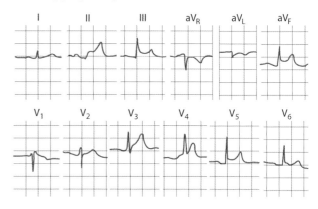

Listening template

Unit 1   page 4

Names

Patient:
Doctor:
Paramedic:

Sequence of events

Place:
Description of the event:
Reaction to the event:
Before the event:
After the event:
Past events:

Student B

Unit 1 p.7

You are the husband / wife of a 50-year-old male / female whom you witnessed collapsing at the entrance to a cinema. The onset was sudden; there was pallor and sweating, rapid recovery, flushing, no nausea, arrhythmia, no incontinence; several similar episodes previously.

Add any further information from your own medical knowledge.

Possible diagnosis: cardiac syncopal event, but need to rule out other possibilities.

Unit 3 p.23

Your notes

> *45 years of age male / female, knee / upper leg, runner, pavement ankle hard roads can't stop has to run, lower back as well / training for marathon*
>
> *audible pop*

Unit 5 p.42

You are Mrs Chaplin. You gave birth to a baby ten days ago. You present to the GP's surgery with a little bit of tearfulness which has gone on longer than the first few days after giving birth. You are getting no support from your friends and family and you are feeling panicky. You

- don't laugh at things as per normal
- look forward to things, but definitely less than before
- know things not your fault even if get on top of you but sometimes reproach yourself
- are often anxious / worried
- are sometimes panicky, but more than normal
- are not coping well
- have problems sleeping
- are miserable a lot of the time
- cried a little first few days then it got worse
- are unhappy and crying a lot
- have never thought of harming self or the baby.

Unit 7 p.69

Choose one of the pictures and show it to the doctor at the appropriate moment.

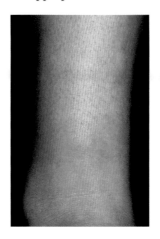 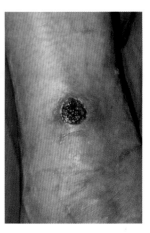

Unit 9 p.85

You are a 40-year-old patient who presents with atrial fibrillation. You are anxious and have a slight chest pain with palpitations and dyspnoea. You fainted before you came to the hospital.

At the appropriate point show the doctor the ECG.

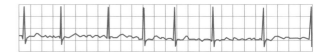

Speaking checklist

Date:	**Candidate:**	
Criteria	Grade*	Comments
1		
2		
3		
4		
5		

*Grades

A Good
B Satisfactory
C Needs improvement

Grammar reference

Unit 1

Rapid tense change

When describing a series of actions, it is very important to convey accurately the sequence of events. It is helpful to remember that the Past Continuous and Past Perfect Continuous provide a background to other actions.

Past Continuous: *I was lifting a box ...*
= Subject + Past Simple of *be* + *-ing* form

Past Perfect Continuous: *My mother had been feeling dizzy for a few days.*
= Subject + Past Simple of *have* + *been* + *-ing* form

We often use the Past Simple for events that interrupt other actions or which are connected to a context that has been provided.

Past Simple: *I was lifting a box when I fell over.*
My mother fainted this morning. She had been feeling dizzy for a few days.

It is common to use the Past Simple to describe a series of consecutive events. We often use words such as *suddenly* and *then* to provide continuity.

I got on the bus and then I sat down. Suddenly, I felt sick.

We use the Past Perfect to refer back to an earlier action that is finished.

Past Perfect: *My father had fallen earlier that day.*
= Subject + Past Simple of *have* + past participle

We use the Present Perfect to talk about something that happened at any time in the past up to the present moment.

Present Perfect: *She hasn't eaten anything today.*
= Subject + Present Simple of *have* + past participle

We use the Present Perfect Continuous to talk about something that has happened continuously or repetitively from a point in the past right up to the present. Sometimes, we can use either a Present Perfect or a Present Perfect Continuous form. The important thing to remember is that the latter emphasizes the continuous aspect of the action.

Present Perfect Continuous: *She's been having dizzy spells for some time now.*
= Subject + Present Simple of *have* + *been* + *-ing* form

We can use time markers such as *when* or *after* to link actions. Be very careful about the tense you use.

*I was cleaning the windows **when** I slipped and broke my leg.* or ***When** I was cleaning the windows, I slipped and broke my leg.*

NOT ~~I cleaned the windows when I slipped and broke my leg.~~

***After** I had rested, I felt better.*
*He doesn't remember anything **after** the ambulance arrived.*

Note the use of the comma when *after* or *when* come at the beginning of the sentence.

Comparative and superlative adjectives and adverbs

Comparative and superlative adjectives

		Adjective	Comparative	Superlative
Short adjective	+ *-er* / *-est*	short	short**er**	the short**est**
Adjective ending in *-e*	+ *-r* / *-st*	large	larg**er**	the larg**est**
Short adjective ending in vowel + consonant, except *-w*	double the consonant + *-er* / *-est*	wet	wet**ter**	the wet**test**
Adjective of two or more syllables	*more* / *most* + adjective	modern	**more** modern	the **most** modern
		expensive	**more** expensive	the **most** expensive
Adjective ending in consonant + *-y*	change *-y* to *-i* + *-er* / *-est*	lively	livel**ier**	the livel**iest**
Irregular adjective		good	better	best
		bad	worse	worst
		far	farther / further	farthest / furthest

Comparative adjectives

We use *than* after the adjective when directly comparing two things.

*In the UK, this treatment is **more expensive than** in the USA.*

We can also use *less* + adjective to mean the opposite of *more*.

*The injury is **less serious** than we thought.*
NOT ~~*The injury is less seriouser ...*~~

We use *more* and *less* before nouns. Note that it is more correct to use *fewer* rather than *less* before countable nouns.

*There is **more information** available now, and **more people** expect a full explanation.*

*In the past, there was **less information** available, and **fewer people** expected a full explanation.*

We use *(not) as ... as* to describe two things or situations that are (not) the same as each other.

*The outcome is **as good as** it possibly can be.*
*The medication is**n't as strong as** the one you were taking before.*

Superlative adjectives

We don't use *than* after a superlative adjective.

*Rest is **the best** treatment we can offer him.*

The superlative forms of *more* and *less* are *the most* and *the least*.

*This is **the most serious** case I've seen.*
*That hospital has **the least up-to-date** facilities in the region.*

Comparative adverbs

We can use *more, less* and *(not) as ... as* in the same way for adverbs as for adjectives.

*She is shaking **more violently** now.*
*He is bleeding **less profusely** than before.*
*Mr Janssen's heart is**n't** beating **as fast as** it was thirty minutes ago.*

We generally don't use adverbs in the superlative form.

Unit 2

Talking about the present

There are several ways to talk about actions in the present or recent past.

Present Perfect

We use the Present Perfect to talk about something that has happened recently. We sometimes use *just* to emphasize a very recent event.

*The patient **has** (just) **discharged** himself.*

*You **haven't broken** your arm.*

= *have / has* (+ *not*) + past participle

We also use the Present Perfect to refer to a time span from any time in the past up to the present.

*He'**s broken** his arm several times.*

= during his life

*She'**s fallen** over twice this month.*

Present Continuous

We use the Present Continuous to describe an action or situation that is happening now. We don't generally use the Present Continuous with verbs of perception such as *think, know, sound* or *look* + adjective.

*My head'**s throbbing**.*
*I'**m getting** pains in my shoulder.*

*His arm **isn't aching** as much as it was before.*

= *am / is / are /* (+ *not*) + *-ing* form

Present Simple

We use the Present Simple to describe a state. We can use the verb *be* or a verb of perception, or verbs such as *need* or *have got*.

*The wound **is** very sore.*
*It **looks** serious.*
*That **doesn't sound** good.*
*He **needs** stronger painkillers.*

We can also use the Present Simple to talk about a habit or repeated action. This is sometimes combined with an adverb of frequency such as *often* or *regularly*.

*She **falls** over very easily.*
*He **doesn't take** his medication every day.*
***Do** you **get** pains in your back?*

With some verbs, we can use either the Present Continuous or Present Simple with no real change in meaning, e.g. *hurt, show,* or *work*.

*It **hurts** just here.*
= *It**'s hurting** just here.*

*The X-ray **shows** a hairline fracture.*
= *The X-ray**'s showing** a hairline fracture.*

*The tablets **don't work**.*
= *The tablets **aren't working**.*

Saying what's necessary politely but firmly

To give a polite instruction, we often use *You need to* + infinitive. This is less direct, and therefore more polite, than using the imperative on its own.

***You need to take** a course of tablets.*
NOT ~~*Take a course of tablets.*~~

We can use the negative form of *need* to say that something isn't necessary.

***You don't need to make** the appointment yourself.*

However, we do use the affirmative and negative imperative as part of an instruction, for example combined with an *if*-clause.

***Ask** your GP **if you're concerned**.* or ***If you're concerned, ask** your GP.*

***Don't wait** for the pain to get worse **before contacting** your doctor again.*

The expression *Don't hesitate to* + infinitive without *to* is a fixed phrase and indicates a desire to be helpful.

***Don't hesitate to call** me.*

Other structures we use with an *if*-clause or other context are *You have to / You must* + infinitive without *to*. On their own, they are much too direct.

***If** the pain gets worse, **you must / have to** let us know immediately.*

Alternative ways of making a direct instruction sound more polite, or of making unwelcome information sound more acceptable, are *You're going to have to / You'll have to / You'll need to* + infinitive without *to*.

***You're going to have to be** admitted, I'm afraid.*
***He'll have to wait** some time for a bed.*

Unit 3

Types of questions

We use different types of questions according to the kind of information we want.

Yes / no questions

These are closed questions. They don't begin with a question word, and generally require a 'yes' or 'no' answer. With yes/no questions, we invert the subject and verb.

***Have you got** the medication with you?*
***Is your knee** painful?*
***Do you take** your medication every day?*
***Can you** bend your arm?*

Wh- questions

When we need to have more information, we ask open questions, often beginning with a question word such as *where, what, when, how, why*. The word order is the same as for yes/no questions.

***What's** the problem?*
***Where** does it hurt?*
***How long** has your leg been infected?*

However, we can modify these questions to make them even more open. We can invite someone to talk about or describe something by using *Can you tell me ...?* or *What do you think ...?*

***Can you tell me** how it happened?*
***What do you think** the problem is?*

Note that in the sentences above, the question form is indirect.

NOT ~~*Can you tell me what is the problem?*~~

We can use a word such as *else* in yes/no or wh-questions to elicit a longer reply from a patient. Note the position of *else*.

***Does it hurt** anywhere **else**?*
***Where else** does it hurt?*
***Is there anything else** you'd like to talk about?*

Unit 4

Giving advice and talking about expectation

There are several ways of talking about the best thing to do in a situation. We generally use modal verbs, which are followed by infinitive without *to*.

Possibility

We use *can* and *may* to talk about possibility.

*Eating certain types of cheese in pregnancy **can/may** be dangerous.*

In the question form, we tend to only use *can*, as *may* is used more commonly when requesting permission.

***Can** drinking raw milk affect the baby?*

Permission

We also use both *can* and *may* to request permission.

*You **can/may** continue to play most sports.*

In the question form, we use *may* to ask about a specific request, such as opening a window. We use *can* when we are asking about a general situation.

***Can** I drink any alcohol during pregnancy?*
but ***May** I have a glass of water, please?*

Necessity

We usually talk about necessity by using the verb *need* + infinitive.

*You'll find you **need** to rest more frequently.*
***Do** I **need** to start taking folic acid now?*

Obligation

Obligation is a stronger form of necessity. We generally use *must/mustn't* and *have to* to talk about obligation.

*Pregnant women **must/ have to** take every opportunity to put their feet up.*

*You **mustn't** do anything that risks raising your blood pressure further.*

Note that the question form of *must* is *Must* + subject, but it is more common to use *Do* + subject + *have to*.

***Do** I **have to** have a special diet?*
NOT ~~*Must I have a special diet?*~~

Persuasion

As a form of advice, we use *should/shouldn't* and

ought to to try to persuade someone to do something.

*You **should** eat more fruit and vegetables.*
*You **ought to** attend all the antenatal appointments if you can.*

*You **shouldn't** try to do too much housework.*

We can also use the negative question form *Can't* as a persuasive device.

Can't I have an appointment sooner?
Can't you refer me to a different clinic?

Note that we often use negative question forms when we are (or want to sound) less certain about something.

***Shouldn't** I be taking any other supplements?*

***Can't** exercise be harmful to the baby?*

Expectation

We also use *should/shouldn't* and *ought to* to talk about expectation.

*You **should/ought to** be careful about drinking too much caffeine.*

*You **shouldn't** have more than three cups of coffee per day.*

Conclusion

We use *must* or *can't* to come to a conclusion or make a deduction.

*An epidural **must** be quite painful, surely?*

*I **can't** be more than six weeks pregnant.*

Unit 5

Phrasal verbs – separable and inseparable

Phrasal verbs are verbs used with different particles which change the meaning of the verb, e.g. *get in* and *get over*. The meaning of these two phrasal verbs is easy to understand. Some phrasal verbs are more idiomatic, so the combination of verb + particle gives a special meaning, e.g. *get over* also means 'recover'.

Some phrasal verbs have an object. Often, the verb and the particle are separable.

*The surgeon **put on** his gloves.*
*The surgeon **put** his gloves **on**.*

However, a pronoun always goes before the particle.

*He **took them off** again.*

NOT   ~~He took off them again.~~

With some phrasal verbs, the verb and particle can't be separated. This depends entirely on the meaning of the phrasal verb. For example:

> *get someone down*

= depress someone

NOT   ~~get down someone~~

> *get down the stairs*

= walk down the stairs

NOT   ~~get the stairs down~~

but

> *get some food down*

= eat some food

These phrasal verbs have to be learnt individually.

Unit 6

would, used to, get used to, be used to

would

We use *would* + infinitive without *to* to talk about a habitual or regular action in the past.

*When I worked at the hospital, I **would** often **take** the train because the parking was so bad.*

*He **would get through** a packet of cigarettes a day.*

We can use the negative form *wouldn't*.

*When she was alive, she **wouldn't** answer the phone unless she was expecting a call.*

used to

We use *used to* + infinitive to talk about habitual or regular actions in the past.

*When I was doing an early shift, I **used to have** breakfast at the hospital.*

*She **used to eat** two chocolate bars every day.*

We can also use *used to* + infinitive to talk about a state or continuous action in the past.

*He **used to be** a heavy smoker.*
NOT   ~~He would be a heavy smoker.~~

*They **used to work** in my department.*
NOT   ~~They would work in my department.~~

The negative form is *didn't use to*.

*There **didn't use to be** a direct bus from here to the hospital.*

get used to

We use *get used to* + noun or *-ing* form to talk about becoming accustomed to a person, thing, or situation. We can use *get used to* in any tense, and form the negative accordingly.

*He's **getting used to** the new rota at work.*
*They've **got used to** working together.*
*I **won't get used to** living in a city very easily.*
*She **can't get used to** these new uniforms.*

be used to

We use *be used to* + noun or *-ing* form to mean that we are accustomed to a person, thing, or situation. We also use *be used to* in different tenses.

*We're **used to** a more dynamic environment.*
*She **won't be used to** running such a large department.*

Purpose and reason

We use *to* and *in order to* before a clause that explains a purpose or gives a reason. *In order to* is often regarded as being more formal than *to* and can carry more emphasis when the opening clause is long. However, in many cases, they can be used interchangeably.

*You need to take regular exercise **to** / **in order to** improve your general fitness.*

*I'll give you a prescription for some tablets **to** / **in order to** help ease the pain.*

Note that *to* / *in order to* must be followed by the infinitive without *to*. We can't introduce a pronoun.

NOT   You need to take regular exercise ~~to / in order to it will improve~~ ...

NOT   You need to take regular exercise ~~to / in order to you will get better.~~

Unit 7

Commenting on the past

We often use the conditional perfect form *would have* + past participle to talk about situations in the past happening differently. In informal language, we sometimes use the contracted form of *have*.

I **would've gone** to see the doctor sooner, but I was on holiday.

It **wouldn't have made** much difference.

We can use other verbs in this structure:

must have

● to talk about deduction
  *She never picked up her prescription. She **must've got** better.*

can't have

● to talk about a negative deduction
  *There are still patients waiting. Doctor Jarvin **can't have left** already.*

could/couldn't have

● to talk about possibility in the past or a lack of opportunity in the past
  *It's just as well the notes mention her allergy. She **could have been** taken seriously ill.*
  *I **couldn't have gone** to the hospital that day even if I'd wanted to.*

should/shouldn't have

● to talk about past obligation or to advise on a course of action in the past
  *You **should have asked** for clarification if you had any doubts about your treatment.*
  *They were quite hostile. They **shouldn't have spoken** to you like that.*

needn't have (*didn't need to* + infinitive without *to*)

● to talk about a course of action in the past that wasn't necessary
  *We **needn't have asked** the doctor to explain the condition, as there was a very helpful leaflet.*

Instead of *needn't have*, we can use *didn't need to* + infinitive without *to*.

We **didn't need to ask** the doctor to explain the condition, as there was a very helpful leaflet.

However, the difference is that in the first sentence, *needn't have* suggests that the people did ask the doctor to explain, but it was unnecessary because they later found a leaflet. In the second sentence, *didn't need to* suggests that the people didn't ask for an explanation because they'd already found the leaflet.

Verbs with *to* and *-ing*

Some verbs are followed by the infinitive, and others are followed by the *-ing* form.

Verbs followed by the infinitive:

These include:
agree, arrange, ask, choose, decide, expect, forget, hope, manage, offer, plan, prepare, promise, threaten, want, wish

We **offered to give** the man a lift to the hospital.

He **didn't want to see** a female doctor.

Verbs followed by the *-ing* form

These include:
admit (to), avoid, carry on, consider, deny, dislike, enjoy, finish, give up, imagine, involve, keep (on), mention, practise, regret, remember, risk, suggest

He **denied wasting** the surgery's time.

Pay attention to the position of the negative form. This depends on whether the main verb or subordinate verb is the negative element.

I **regret not telling** my family sooner.

N.B. this is the opposite of I **don't regret telling** my family sooner.

Verbs followed by the infinitive or *-ing* form

There are some verbs that can be followed by either the infinitive or the *-ing* form, with no change in meaning.

These include:
continue, intend, like, love, mean, prefer, start, try

I'll **continue working / to work** here for as long as I can.

They **tried talking / to talk** reasonably to the man, who was being very aggressive.

Unit 8

Relative pronouns in explanations

We often use relative pronouns to connect a series of sentences describing an activity or situation.

These pronouns are *who, which, where,* and *when.* The pronouns *who* and *which* can be replaced by *that.*

Who

- used for people, and can be combined with a preposition
  *The patient, **to who(m)** the consent form will be given, must be sufficiently alert to sign it.*

Which

- refers to things, procedures, or situations. *Which* can also be combined with a preposition.
  *The tube is then connected, **which** enables the patient to breathe normally.*
  *The patient is connected to a monitoring device, **to which** other tubes are attached.*
  *This is a procedure **in which** we remove part of the bowel.*

Where

- = 'in which'. We use *where* to talk about what is involved in a procedure or situation.
  *This is an operation **where** we remove part of the bowel.*

When

- = 'after which time' or 'at which point'. *When* describes a point in a sequence of events at which something is expected to occur.
  *The anaesthetic is reduced and the patient taken to the recovery room, **when** he or she will start to come round.*

Sometimes, we can omit the relative pronoun and have a participle as a connector. This is common when we are connecting more than two clauses, to avoid having a sentence that is too long and clumsy.

This is a complex procedure. It is performed under general anaesthetic.
*This is a complex procedure, **performed** under general anaesthetic.* (= 'which is performed')
We're going to do a procedure which will involve major surgery.
*We're going to do a procedure **involving** major surgery.* (= 'which will involve')

Unit 9

The future

There are several different ways of talking about the future.

will

We use *will* to talk about the future in general.
*The presentation **will finish** at about 4 o'clock.*
*There **won't be** much time for questions afterwards.*

We can also use *will* in the main clause of a first conditional sentence.
If the presentation finishes earlier, there'll be more time for questions.

Present Simple

We use the Present Simple to talk about the future in the *if*-clause of a first conditional sentence.

We also use the Present Simple to talk about future timetabled events.

*Dr Carlin's train **leaves** London at 1.30 and **gets into** Oxford at 2.10.*

We also use the Present Simple with time expressions such as *before, after, as soon as,* and *when.*

*We need to make sure that everything is ready **before** Dr Carlin arrives.*
NOT *... before Dr Carlin will arrive.*

***When he gets** here, could you let me know?*
NOT *When he will get here ...*

Present Continuous

We use the Present Continuous to talk about something that has been planned or arranged. When this includes timetabled events, it is possible to use either the Present Simple or the Present Continuous.

*The ceremony **is taking** place in November.*
  or *The ceremony **takes** place in November.*

However:

*We're **sending** out invitations over the next couple of weeks.*
NOT *We send out invitations ...*

Future Continuous

We use the Future Continuous to talk about an action that will be happening at a given point in the future. This can be part of a schedule or can be a continuous action. However, this tense must always be used with a time reference.

Will the doctor **be starting** her rounds before 10.30?

This time next week, you'll be flying back to the USA.

= Subject + *will* + *be* + *-ing* form

Future Perfect

We use the Future Perfect to talk about an action that will have finished at a given point in the future.

*Dr Singh **will have finished** his rounds by lunchtime.*

= Subject + *will* + *have* + past participle

Will he **have left** intensive care by then?

Future Perfect Continuous

We use the Future Perfect Continuous to talk about an action that leads up to a given point in the future. The action isn't necessarily finished at that future point.

*This is a long presentation. By five o'clock, Dr Schwartz **will have been talking** for an hour and a half.*

(= it's possible that Dr Schwartz will continue beyond five o'clock)
= Subject + *will* + *have* + *been* + *-ing* form

Unit 10

The definite and indefinite article

The rules for using *the, a, an,* or zero article are as follows:

the

We use the definite article *the* before singular or plural countable nouns when we want to make it clear which person or thing we're referring to.

***The disease** is spreading very quickly.*

(= a specific disease, which we have talked about in a previous sentence)

***The number** of people being admitted to hospital with 'flu has increased dramatically.*

(= a specific quantity)

*Binge drinking is **a major cause** of liver disease.*

(= there are other factors, but we don't know how significant they are)

We use *the* when there is only one of the thing we're talking about.

***The government** is cutting spending on health.*

(= the government of a particular country)

***The sun** is a major source of vitamin D.*

a, an

We use the indefinite articles *a* and *an* before singular countable nouns when it isn't necessary to make clear which particular thing we are talking about.

*We need to make **a** decision about the future of this unit.*

(= any decision)

Compare with:

***The decision** was not very popular.*

(= the decision that was eventually made)

***A number** of people have presented with the same symptoms.*

(= several)

*Binge drinking is **the major cause** of liver disease.*

(= it is a significantly greater factor than other possible causes)

zero article

We use no article (zero article) before plural or uncountable nouns when we are talking about something in general.

***Disease** is a major factor in early mortality in many developing countries.*

(= disease in general)

***People** need to be informed about safe levels of consumption.*

(= people everywhere)

Compare with:

***The people** who drink and smoke to excess are the ones who cost the government most.*

(= a specific group of people)

***Governments** are looking to reduce health costs.*

(= the governments of several or all countries)

Unit 11

Linking words

There are several ways of linking ideas within sentences and between one sentence and the next.

when

When refers to a particular time or stage in a process.

__When__ a person is bitten by the tsetse fly, he or she may experience symptoms such as fever and headaches.

At a later stage, sleeping sickness enters a neurological phase, __when__ the parasite passes through the blood-brain barrier.

where

Where expands on a process or procedure.

In a biopsy, __where__ a sample of tissue is removed for further testing, the patient is often given only a local anaesthetic.

Where can also describe a location.

The camera is inserted into the stomach, __where__ it is able to take images of the lining.

then

Then introduces the next stage in a process or procedure. Look at how the punctuation is used.

__Then__, the parasite enters the blood and lymph systems.

The lymph nodes __then__ swell up.

If left untreated, other symptoms such as anaemia will appear, __and then__ the disease enters a neurological phase.

after that

After that is a general term, signalling the next stage in a process or procedure. There is no indication of how much time has passed between the two stages. Its meaning and use is similar to *then*. We can say *after that happens* to refer more specifically to an action that has just been described.

The disease had practically disappeared between 1969 and 1965. __After that__, screening and surveillance were relaxed and the disease has now returned.

after this

After this is slightly more specific than *after that*, and means more immediately after the last point or stage made. We can also say *after this happens*.

The patient is taken into recovery. __After this__, he or she is returned to the ward.

next

Next is similar to *after that*. However, we tend to use *next* at the beginning of the sentence.

Next, the patient is returned to the ward.

once

Once as a time reference must be followed by a clause. It means that the next stage of the process can't begin until the previous stage is completed. The second stage follows on immediately.

__Once__ the patient __recovers__, he or she is taken back to the ward.

NOT   *Once, the patient starts to recover*

The Present Simple and Present Perfect can be used after *once* with no real difference in meaning.

__Once__ the patient __has recovered__, he or she is taken back to the ward.

as soon as

As soon as is similar to *once* in meaning and use. However, *as soon as* + Present Simple suggests that two stages are happening almost at the same time.

__As soon as__ the patient __comes__ round, let me know.

As soon as + Present Perfect suggests that the first action is completed before the second one begins.

__As soon as__ the doctor __has consulted__ with his colleague, he will speak to you.

Unit 12

Negative questions

We often use negative questions to avoid being overly direct when making a demand or criticism, or when reminding or persuading someone to do something.

The choice of a negative question can suggest that the speaker has expectations and wants to avoid a direct 'yes' or 'no' response. A less direct question can also show that the speaker is trying to avoid criticism. For example, beginning a question *Isn't the consultant going to be talking to my daughter?* is much less assertive than *Is the consultant going to talk to my daughter?*

- The most straightforward type of negative question is one that appears to be requesting information.
  Aren't *these tablets very expensive?*

  The speaker knows that they're expensive and is checking that this is understood. Compare with the more open affirmative question: *Are these tablets very expensive?*

  When we expect something to have happened, we can use the negative form *Haven't / Hasn't.* The addition of *yet* makes this a stronger criticism.

  Haven't they found my records *yet*?

- A question beginning with *Can't* or *Couldn't* is an attempt to persuade a person in a decision-making role to agree to their demand or request. The choice of an affirmative question would risk inviting a 'no' response.
  Can't / Couldn't *I (just) call in and get the results
      myself?*
  An alternative is Wouldn't it be better ...?
  Wouldn't it be better *if I phoned the hospital
      myself?*

- We often convey shock or surprise as well as criticism by beginning a question with *Shouldn't.*
  Shouldn't *you have told us about this sooner?*

  It would not make sense to begin this question with *Should.* The speaker is implying that the other person is acting irresponsibly. We could also use *Couldn't* here, to indicate that it was within another person's capacity to do something.

- To remind someone about something, we can use *Didn't you say ...?* This is followed by an indirect speech clause, but ends in a question mark.
  Didn't you say *that I would be near the top of the
      waiting list?*

Listening scripts

Unit 1

Listening 1

D = Doctor, P = Patient

D Hi, Mr Stone, I'm Dr Tariq, one of the doctors in A&E. How are you?

P I'm OK, but I'm a bit worried about my wife.

D Your wife's OK.

P That's good.

D Amir, one of the paramedics, says you were walking along the street when your wife collapsed. Can you tell me a bit more about what you actually saw?

P Mmm. Yes, sure. We were shopping in Cambridge Street in town, when suddenly Barbara, my wife, just fainted. Mmm, we tried to get her upright and she started twitching quite violently. It was quite scary.

D Yes, it certainly can be, but it can happen when people faint like this. Did anything else happen?

P No. Nothing at all. She came round very rapidly. But we dialled 999 and a paramedic appeared almost instantly and then the ambulance almost immediately afterwards. Do you think she had a seizure or something like epilepsy?

D We don't think so. But can I ask you a few more questions? Did she complain of anything before that?

P Mmm. She had been complaining of feeling a bit unwell, and had almost fainted and she felt a bit woozy? She ... yes, er... she was a bit dizzy and she was yawning repeatedly and then all of a sudden, there she was, lying on the ground.

D Anything else? Was she ill or anything before she fell?

P No. Just tired.

D What about her eyesight?

P Nothing, but she said her hearing was a bit funny – she wasn't hearing clearly.

D Any vomiting?

P No.

D When she fell, how did she fall?

P She just crumpled to the ground slowly. In fact, it all happened so abruptly and silently I didn't realize it had happened.

D So she didn't cry out or anything?

P No, there was no warning sign at all.

D Just a few more questions.

P OK.

D Has she ever had anything like this before?

P When I come to think of it, she passed out once before about a month ago. She hasn't been feeling well off and on over the summer. We thought it was the heat.

D At the moment it looks like ...

Listening 2

Gary Edwards, a British Airways customer service arrivals agent, had been sitting with his work colleagues in a rest room at Heathrow Airport's Terminal One when he suffered severe pain in his chest and arms. Within seconds, he lost consciousness and stopped breathing. His British Airways colleagues immediately dialled 999 for an ambulance and began attempts to resuscitate him.

All he can remember is that he had got up from the sofa and said to his colleagues that his chest and arm hurt. After that, everything went blank. Within seconds of the 999 call being made, cycle paramedic Dave Parks reached Mr Edwards. Dave was able to continue resuscitation and re-start Mr Edwards's heart after three attempts using the portable defibrillator that is carried on ambulance bicycles.

Paramedics, dispatched in an ambulance at the same time as the bicycle ambulance, arrived a few minutes later to continue treatment and took Mr Edwards to hospital. This resuscitation shows how well-suited bikes are to reaching patients quickly inside the airport. As they are based at the airport and were able to get to him so quickly, it most probably made the difference between life and death.

Dave emphasized the importance of quick intervention when someone suffers a cardiac arrest and took the opportunity to remind members of the public that they can learn cardiopulmonary resuscitation – or CPR – at free 'Heartstart' classes given across the capital by the London Ambulance Service and supported by the British Heart Foundation. Effective CPR buys time for a patient and doubles a person's chances of survival.

Unit 2

Listening 1

D = Doctor, P = Patient

1

D You look as if you are in quite a lot of pain.

P Yes, I think I've hurt my hip badly. It's giving me a lot of pain.

D I think we need to get you some painkillers. So ... can you tell me a bit more?

P Oh, I slipped on the kitchen floor. I must have spilled some water and I was coming into the living room with a cup of tea and I just went down on my bottom and twisted my leg.

D Oh, dear. That sounds bad.

P It was. I couldn't move. Fortunately, I had my mobile in my apron pocket and I phoned my neighbour who had the key to come in. She called an ambulance.

D Falls like this happen so easily. You may just have pulled a joint out of place rather than breaking anything.

2

D What's brought you here today?

P My wrist is really hurting. I think I've broken it.

D OK. How did it happen?

P Well, I was coming out of a shop and I was trying to avoid someone and I didn't notice the paving stone was raised and I just tripped and of course I put out my hands to protect myself and break my fall. My wrist took the full force of my fall.

D It certainly looks quite bad, yes. I think we need to do an X-ray.

3

D = Doctor, F = Patient's father

D What's happened here?

F She fell down from a tree at school and they called me and I came here from work as the ambulance was bringing her here.

D Oh, I see.

F She's crying a lot and I think she's fractured something in her leg.

D She may not have broken anything, but let's have a look at her.

Language spot

1 So you've taken some painkillers, but they don't work, and your arm's still hurting you just here.

2 My toe is throbbing with pain. I don't know what I've done. It looks as if it's broken.

3 He's had several falls recently and he has several fractures, but he's not crying a lot.

Listening 2

As health professionals, we give advice about healthy lifestyles, which should include accident prevention. When we use the word *accident*, it seems to imply that accidents are unavoidable. It is true that we do not live a life free of risk, but the danger of accidents can be minimized by simple precautions … and thinking ahead.

We can, for example, make patients aware of the potential for risk. All risk situations including those in the home or garden, in the workplace, on the road, or during leisure activities such as hillwalking or mountain climbing should be treated with due respect. People need to be reminded to think of others, especially children and the elderly. Once an accident has happened

it is too late to go back and take precautions.

There are many simple pieces of advice that can be given to prevent accidents in the home like fitting stairs with banisters or rails and making sure that halls and stairways are well lit. Encouraging people to climb up only on something firm and strong can help reduce the risk of falls. Another thing to avoid is loose rugs and flooring in order to reduce the risk of slipping or tripping especially when old people or children are around. And if small children are about, ponds and swimming pools in the garden need to be covered.

DIY at home or home improvements is another area with potential for accidents. When using power tools, people need to be encouraged to use adequate protection including sturdy shoes, gloves, and goggles.

Unit 3

Listening 1

D = Doctor, P = Patient

Conversation A

D So what has happened to you, Mrs Skinner?

P Well, I've hurt my hand.

D Right. When did it happen?

P I've had it since the week before last.

D Hm, where do you get the pain?

P Here on the heel of my hand.

D Is that both hands?

P No, just this one.

D And have you taken anything for it?

P I've tried painkillers and that, but they haven't worked. When the tablets wear off, it's still there. I don't have a touch of arthritis, do you think?

D At this stage it's difficult to say. It's something we have to try and rule out. But can I just ask you what you think caused it?

P I don't really know.

D Anything at work?

P I don't know. It may be the work. I type a lot.

D OK. So you sit at a desk all day.

P Yes.

D Mm. Now the pain, does it … ?

Conversation B

D So what has happened to you, Mrs Skinner?

P Well, I've hurt my hand.

D Tell me a bit more about it.

P I've had it since the week before last here on the heel of my hand, and I'm finding it difficult to work and also to go to the gym. I've tried painkillers and that, but they haven't worked. When the tablets wear off, it's still there. I don't have a touch of arthritis, do you think?

D At this stage it's difficult to say. It's something we have to try and rule out. But can I just ask you what you think caused it?

P I don't really know. It may be the work.

D Can you tell me when it is worst?

P Mmm. When I'm at the gym, when I'm typing, and when the boss is around!

D Yes, I can imagine the boss making it worse. You mentioned the gym.

P Yes.

D Do you go a lot?

P Yes, I do.

D I'd just like you to put your arm …

Listening 2

D = Doctor, P = Patient

D Alexander, you've had quite a bang on your head.

P Yeah, and I'm surprised I feel OK. I thought it might give me a really bad headache or something, but I really feel fine. I'm just a bit shaken, really.

D Yes. These things can knock you quite a bit. You still need to be careful over the next twenty-four hours, even though you feel fine.

P What? You mean I have to stay in the hospital?

D Oh, no, you don't need to stay in hospital, but we need you to look after yourself and rest for the next twenty-four hours.

P Rest? But I can't. I have to go to my best friend's party this evening. I just can't miss it. He's getting married tomorrow.

D But I'm afraid you do need to be careful. And you need to have someone to go home with you and stay with you for the next twenty-four hours as well.

P But I feel OK. I mean, why all the fuss?

D Yes, you may feel well, but some things may develop afterwards.

P Like what?

D You may get a headache.

P Well, I can take a paracetamol.

D Yes, but other things could happen like blurred vision or vomiting.

P OK, but I can come back if anything goes wrong.

Pronunciation

1 Can you tell me a little bit more about how it all happened?

2 But if your child's mood changes in any way, make sure you contact us immediately.

3 But I can't. I have to go to my best friend's party this evening.

4 But I'm afraid you do need to be careful.

5 I'm not sure but I think I've torn a ligament in my foot. It's swollen and I can't get my shoe on.

6 I've had it since the week before last, here on the heel of my hand.

7 And you need to have someone to go home with you and stay with you for the next twenty-four hours as well.

Unit 4

Listening

D = Doctor, P = Patient

Exercise 4

D Good morning, Mrs Canterbury. How are you enjoying this fine weather we're having?

P I love it. It's been the best we've had for a long time.

D Yes, it's been remarkable. Let's hope it continues.

P Well, I think it may.

D Yes. It looks like it. So, what can we do for you?

P Mmm, well, doctor, it's not really trouble, I think … I think I'm expecting.

D Ah, I see, and are you happy about that?

P Oh, yes, we've been trying for ages.

D OK. Well, let's take some details. Can you remember when your last period was?

P Mmm, not exactly, but probably about six weeks ago.

D So you think you've missed one?

P Yes. I'm as regular as clockwork.

D Any other changes you've noticed?

P Er, I do feel a bit sick most mornings, and my breasts feel a bit tender.

D Right, if I give you a little bowl, can you just pop to the toilet and bring back a sample for me?

Exercise 5

D Well, congratulations, Mrs Canterbury, you were right, you are expecting, and if your dates are correct you're probably about four weeks gone.

P Oh, so the baby'll probably be born in October.

D Around then, yes. We'll be able to be more precise after you've had a scan.

P When will that be?

D It's usually done at about twelve weeks. By that time we can usually get a clear picture of the baby. Now, I take it you'll have your baby in hospital?

P I haven't really thought about it.

D Well since it's your first, it's probably best. We'll check your details later and sort out the hospital.

P So you'll let me know which hospital it'll be?

D Yes, that's right. Now I just want to ask you a few questions about your lifestyle. Do you eat sensibly?

P Generally yes, though I do skip meals sometimes when I'm rushed.

D Well, it's very important now that you make sure you eat nutritious food regularly.

P I realize that. Um, does it matter what I eat?

D Yes, there are certain things you need to steer clear of, like shellfish and soft cheese. You don't want to risk any kind of food poisoning. Now what about alcohol?

P A couple of glasses now and then, but I haven't been on a binge for ages.

D Good, well keep it that way. Alcohol should really be avoided in pregnancy, but the occasional drink will do no harm. Do you smoke?

P Occasionally, but it's not a real habit.

D Well, try to cut down, if not give up altogether. With a growing baby inside you, you need to be very careful what you are putting into your body. Are there any questions you'd like to ask?

P No.

D And congratulations, Mrs Canterbury.

P Thank you very much.

Pronunciation

1 At vaginal hysterectomy, the uterus is brought down through the vagina.

2 What happens is the womb is brought down through the vagina.

3 Pre-eclampsia is pregnancy-induced hypertension with proteinuria with or without oedema.

4 It's a condition where the blood pressure is raised with protein in the urine and possibly swelling.

5 Normal labour is often heralded by a show.

6 When an induction is being planned, the state of the cervix will be assessed.

7 Ankle swelling is very common when you're pregnant.

8 It tends to worsen at night? Well, if you use a firm mattress and wear flat shoes, it will help.

Unit 5

Listening 1

He's Caucasian, around about fifty years of age. His clothes are very extravagant with lots of clashing bright colours. But he is not very clean in himself, and he doesn't look as if he's eating properly. It's the first time that I've seen the patient, but he looks just a little thin.

He's not very aggressive, just elated and is talking rather fast. There is copious rapid speech, which is hard to interrupt. He talks at a much faster rate than normal, which may reflect the acceleration of speed of thought in affective illnesses. The patient stutters slightly and speaks rather loudly.

His speech has a rhythmic pattern and he uses a range of intonation patterns appropriately. The speech is appropriate to the situation, though it is fast. It is at times pointless with digressions.

There are no word-finding difficulties nor any neologisms.

Pronunciation

1 I can laugh at the problems I have.
2 It's difficult to distinguish one day from another at the moment.
3 Of course I care for the child.
4 I'm not trying to hint at anything.
5 She insisted on going home.
6 I sometimes blame myself for the day-to-day problems.
7 The child depends on me for everything.

Listening 2

D = Doctor, P = Patient

D Now, I want to ask you about some experiences which sometimes people have but find it difficult to talk about. These are questions I ask everyone. Is that OK?

P Yeah.

D Have you ever had the sensation that you were unreal or that the world had become unreal?

P It's like ... I don't know how to explain it. It's ... I suppose it's like being in a play somehow. That maybe sounds as if I'm going mad.

D Have you ever had the experience of hearing noises or voices when there was no one there to explain it?

P Yes, sometimes.

D Is it OK to talk about this further?

P Yeah, if you want.

D When did it happen?

P The last time was a couple of days ago.

D Were you fully awake?

P Yeah, it was during the day.

D How often has it happened?

P Recently only once or twice.

D And where did the sound appear to come from?

P I don't know. From someone in the room.

Unit 6

Listening 1

1

M = Man, D = Doctor

M She used to be able to get around quite easily. In fact, she would often go out all over the place in the bus. And I think she finds it difficult getting used to the changes in her life. But now she says that she gets a bit muzzy in the head when she's standing at times and then when she manages to sit down it all passes.

D Has she fallen at all?

M Mmm, yes. Sometimes she doesn't make it to a chair and her legs give way and down she goes. I don't know how she hasn't hurt herself at all.

2

M = Man, W = Woman

M It was really exciting, the whole experience. But I'm not sure I'd want to go through it that often.

W How many people were there?

M Five or six others, I think. They were very high calibre. A couple of them had years of experience working in care of the elderly. One used to run a geriatric hospital in his own country. I don't think I stood a chance.

3

W = Woman, M = Man

W There are a couple of things that could be done to help this patient. We could get in occupational health to get things like a perching stool installed and grab rails.

M Yes, and also flooring and lighting. And I don't think all the clutter helps. As the place is full of rubbish, small changes like that will help a lot.

4

D = Doctor, C = Consultant

D And apart from the expression there are other tell-tale signs like difficulty in swallowing, a decrease in the blink rate, and lead-pipe rigidity.

C Did you pick up anything else with this patient?

D Mmm ... the handwriting.

C What about it?

D It was really small. His wife said in the past he would write very long elegant letters and now ...

Listening 2

D = Doctor, P = Patient

D Can you tell me how it affects you, Mrs Day?

P I don't know where to start. I feel tired a lot of the time because the pain keeps me awake at night. And at work I can't sit for long. I have to get up and walk around. At work, people don't know how bad it is and it upsets me when they make comments.

D Unfortunately, unless people have things like this themselves, they don't realize how bad it is.

P No, I'm afraid not.

D Is there anything else?

P Mmm ... it stops me doing certain things ... like I can't catch the bus, because I'm afraid of falling if the bus suddenly jolts, and I can't really go out and enjoy myself.

D What about the tablets your GP prescribed? Have you been taking them?

P Not really. Sometimes.

D Sometimes.

P Yeah.

D Can you tell me why that is?

P I don't like taking them in case I get hooked or anything like that or in case they affect my stomach.

D But when you do take them, do they help?

P Yes, for a while. When the pain is so bad I can't bear it, I take them.

D So you take them when the pain's intolerable.

P Yeah.

D Have you been doing any physiotherapy?

P No, not really.

D What about exercise?

P When I start to do anything it hurts a lot. So it puts me off.

D Well, you know, to help improve your strength and build up your muscles, exercise like swimming really helps.

Unit 7

Listening 1

D = Doctor, P = Patient

D Good morning, John. How are you today?

P Fine, doctor, except for the weather!

D Yes, it's a bit uncomfortable at the moment. We're not used to the heat. We want it, but when we get it, we can't cope.

P Yes, you're right there. We're never happy.

D So what can we do for you?

P Well, I've got this rash with big wheals all over. And it's quite itchy and getting worse.

D Oh, yes. It does look quite dramatic. Can you tell me some more about it?

P Well, I just suddenly came out in it last night. It started on my back and then it just spread. I put some lotion on it, and it helped for a while ... and then I thought *they are getting so bad, I'm itching all over.* And with the heat it's unbearable.

D So you have them everywhere? OK, we'll have a look in a moment. But can you just tell me ... you said you used a lotion?

P Calamine lotion. It was all I had, and then this morning I came straight here.

D You said itching. Is there any pain with it?

P No, just itching.

D OK, just itching. Have you had it before?

P Yes, once I had it, and I came here and they gave me some antihistamine, and it went away, but it wasn't as bad as this. I should've kept the name of the tablets or kept some as they helped before. They just seem to be spreading all over.

D Were the tablets Piriton?

P Yes, I think they were.

D OK. Is there anything you think that might have triggered this?

P Not that I'm aware of.

D Pets?

P I don't have a pet, and I haven't been near any.

D What about drugs?

P No, I'm not on anything.

D Are you aware of being allergic to anything?

P No, I don't think so.

Listening 2

D = Doctor, P = Patient

D OK, thank you. You can put your shirt back on again.

P OK.

D From what I can see it's acne.

P Can you do anything for it?

D Oh, yes.

P That's a relief.

D Has this been upsetting you?

P Yes, a little.

D Can you tell me how?

P I get teased at college about it, and I don't like going out as people look at it ... and I think it's dirty. And it keeps getting worse. I've tried cutting out certain foods, but nothing works, and using different creams and stuff.

D Well, I can assure, it's nothing to do with being dirty. And it's more common than you think. You are nearly seventeen now?

P Yeah.

D Well, the peak age is about eighteen. And diet doesn't affect acne either.

P Ah, OK.

D But the creams you've been using might just make it worse.

P Mmm, yeah, I shouldn't have used them. I should've come here.

D Yes, but you're here now – that's the main thing.

P Yeah.

D So what we need to do first is to reduce the number of spots.

P OK.

D Acne's nothing to do with poor hygiene, but if you wash twice a day and then put on a moisturizer like aqueous cream, that will help.

P Aque ...

D Aqueous cream. It's this. It comes in tubs like this. And cream here. I'm going to give you some cream – benzoyl peroxide – to put on twice a day and this antibiotic cream. I take it you are not taking antibiotic tablets or capsules.

P No, I'm not.

D Now, I must point out that these can take weeks to work, so you need to be patient.

P But they will go away?

D We will certainly do our best to make sure they do. Do you think you'll be able to keep going with the treatment?

P I think so.

D Would you like to see the nurse who can go through it with you?

P Yeah.

D And I'm going to give you this print out from an acne support group. It's got their website on it. You can check it out.

P OK, thanks.

D So you think you'll be OK with this?

P Yeah, I feel better.

D OK. You can take this prescription and make an appointment to see the nurse and come back and see me in a couple of months, but if you need to come back sooner, by all means do.

Pronunciation

1 I should've kept on using the cream you gave me.

2 I should've taken it all more seriously.

3 I have to say I regret not applying the cream now.

4 I shouldn't have put anything on it as that's what's made it worse.

5 I meant to get up and do it first thing in the morning but I didn't.

6 I must've picked it and made it bleed.

7 I stopped using it because it made my skin itchy.

Unit 8

Pronunciation

1 laparotomy
2 nephrectomy
3 colostomy
4 hysterectomy
5 thoracoplasty
6 mastopexy
7 cystorrhaphy
8 cholecystectomy
9 pyelolithotomy
10 colopexy

Listening 1

D = Doctor, P = Patient

D Good afternoon, Mr Blackstone. My name is Dr Petrov. How are you today?

P Fine, thank you, doctor.

D You're coping with all this rain we're having?

P Yeah. It's a bit much at the moment.

D Yes, it's slowing down everything. Right. I see from your GP's letter that you've got a hernia. Am I right?

P Mmm. Yes. I've got this swelling in my groin.

D OK. Can you tell me about it?

P It's just down here in my groin on the right side. It's been there for about three or four months now. It's a bit uncomfortable when it is sticking out; I'm aware of it. I try to sort of put it back in, but it only happens when I'm lying down. I'm a ... I'm a driver so I sometimes have to do a lot of lifting and that.

D You said the hernia pops back in again when you're lying down?

P Yes.

D Has there ever been any time when it's stayed out?

P No, though sometimes it takes its time going back in again.

D Hm, right. OK. Shall we have a look?

P OK.

...

D OK, as your GP says, you've got what is called an inguinal hernia.

P Mm-hm.

D Do you know what a hernia is exactly?

P Not really.

D You can get a hernia like you have where there is a weakness in the membrane or the lining that holds in all the gut. Part of the gut then sticks out at the weak point and forms a bulge, which is what has happened here. Let me just draw it for you.

P OK. I ... I see. Can you fix it?

D Yes. We can do an operation called a herniorrhaphy, where we repair the weak part of the gut using a special mesh. What we do is make one or two small holes in your tummy, one around the belly button and the other on the left side. It's a day-case surgery, so you'll be in and out quite quickly. How do you feel about having the operation?

P Oh, yeah, no problem. Will I be put to sleep?

D Well, we can do this under a local anaesthetic or general.

P I don't fancy being awake and hearing and seeing everything.

D Yes, I can understand why you wouldn't want that. It can be a bit off-putting to some people, but we'll see what the anaesthetist has to say when he does the assessment. Er, we'll need you to sign a consent form if you're happy with everything when you come for a pre-operation assessment.

P Yeah. I'm OK with that.

D Is there anything you'd like to ask me?

P Mmm, er, what about the pain?

D We can talk about the pain at the assessment.

Listening 2

D = Doctor, P = Patient

1

D Would you like me to go over anything again?

P No, I don't think so.

D Do you feel OK about signing the form?

P I'm not sure. I'm a bit worried about what might happen afterwards. It's a big step and a bit drastic. I'm ... I'm not sure I want to go through with it.

D Would you like some time to think about it and perhaps talk to other women who've had their womb removed?

2

P Can't you squeeze me in at all today? This is the second time this has happened.

D I'm afraid we can't. There's an emergency, and there're no beds available.

P But the same thing happened the last time.

D Unfortunately, yes, it did, but the situation's unavoidable.

P OK. Can you guarantee this won't happen the next time?

3

P Will they come back?

D I'm afraid we can't guarantee they won't.

P Is it common?

4

D I can see you're a bit apprehensive about this.

P I am, yes.

D What are you worried about in particular?

P Well, a number of things. Feeling pain, seeing what's going on, hearing everything, and the smell. If I'm awake, will I feel any pain?

D No. You won't feel any pain, but you'll feel your insides being touched.

P And what about seeing what's happening?

5

A = Anaesthetist, P = Patient

A Have you had a general anaesthetic before?

P Yes.

A Recently?

P No, not for a couple of years.

A Did you have any problems with the anaesthetic?

P No, nothing. But I don't like having general anaesthetics.

Unit 9

Listening 1

W = Patient's wife, D = Doctor

W He's not very well at all, is he doctor?

D He's actually OK. He's a bit more stable.

W That's a relief.

D I just need to ask you a few quick questions. Can you tell me what happened?

W We were sitting at home and he started getting this pain in the centre of his chest. He'd had it several times before and he used the spray thing he's got.

D The GTN spray?

W Yeah ... yeah that's it. And so he gave himself a few puffs but the pain wouldn't go and I could see that he was getting breathless and agitated and he said he felt sick. He started vomiting a little ... and he was beginning to sweat. And he said he thought he was going to die.

D OK. So can you tell me what time that was?

W Well, I called for an ambulance at sevenish and it came like a shot, ... so it was less than an hour ago in total.

D So has he had any other pain?

W He said the pain was in both arms.

...

D Your husband is doing very well. It's good you got him straight into hospital, but I need to ask you a few quick questions.

W OK.

D Has your husband had any injuries or any other major illness?

W No.

D Any bleeding?

W No.

D Any major surgery?

W No, nothing like that.

D Anything else you can think of?

W No. Nothing.

D OK. What we're going to need to do, with your consent, is to give your husband something to help get rid of any blood clots. There is a risk of stroke with the procedure, and ...

... but the benefit can be dramatic if we get it down quickly. It can have a considerable effect. There doesn't seem to be any reason why he shouldn't have the medication, but we need to give it as soon as possible and we need your consent.

W OK. Can I just ask ...

...

D By the looks of it, it's all gone very well and he'll be up and about in no time. For the moment he just needs a bit of rest.

Pronunciation

1 He'll have been in the theatre for over three hours in a few minutes' time.

2 Dr Nur isn't starting his clinic till two p.m.

3 He'll be in and out in no time.

4 All being well, he'll be able to go home by the weekend.

5 The operation's scheduled for five this afternoon.

6 You're having the veins on the right leg stripped this afternoon, am I right?

7 The doctor said I'll be having a general anaesthetic.

8 He'll have been coming to the clinic off and on for the past three years.

Listening 2

D = Doctor, P = Patient

D OK, Mary. Your blood pressure is quite high, one-forty over eight-five. I think the last time it was fairly normal.

P Yes, it was. That was about a year ago.

D Mmm, it was a year ago last July.

P At least I've been healthy all this time, apart from these headaches.

D Yes. Well, everything else seems to be OK, so there may be no other cause. I'll run a few tests just to make sure that your kidneys, etc. are OK and we can refer you for an ECG at the hospital.

P OK.

D Is there anything you think might be the cause of the high blood pressure?

P Well, since I took early retirement I've been less active and I've put on quite a bit of weight. I used to be quite active, but I've let things slip a little.

D So when did you retire?

P About a year and a half ago.

D Do you know how much you weigh now?

P Mmm, I weighed myself about two weeks ago and I was a hundred and twelve kilos which for my height I think is quite heavy, I know.

D OK, let's just check your weight and height.

...

D For your height, which is five foot eleven inches, or about one point eight metres, your weight which is now a hundred and fifteen kilos is quite high, if you look on this chart – it should be somewhere here.

P Oh. That is quite a lot over. I do need to get it down.

D Yes. I see from your family history, your father had heart problems and there's a family history of heart disease.

P Yes, on my father's side, all his brothers and sisters had problems with angina.

D If nothing shows up in the tests, you seem to be generally quite healthy, but the problem is hypertension, which can lead to other problems.

P Mmm, I'm aware of that.

D Do you think you can get your weight down easily?

P I can try. Well I just have to … somehow.

D Did you do any sport before?

P Well, I used to swim and walk a lot.

D Have you thought of starting up again?

P Yeah, I suppose I could.

D You'll feel the benefit of it quite quickly and if you're careful with what you eat, you'll be back to what you were before.

P I hope so.

D Would you like to …

Unit 10

Vocabulary

Coughs: 1 dry, 2 hoarse, 3 barking, 4 productive, 5 wheezy

Listening 1

D = Doctor, P = Patient

P I've got this really bad cough, doctor, and I can't shake it off.

D OK. So the cough's been getting worse. Tell me a little bit more about it.

P Well, I've had this cough for a week or so, and it's been getting worse. I didn't think anything of it as I tend to get something at this time of year. But it's there all the time and the phlegm I bring up – it's a greenish-yellow colour and it's streaked with blood. And I have a touch of fever.

D You said the phlegm was streaky?

P Yes, but only a little.

D And how much phlegm do you produce?

P Not that much. It would be less than a teaspoon each time.

D So not much.

P No. And it comes up quite easily. I try to get it up to try and keep my chest clear.

D And is there any smell?

P No. Not that I've noticed. It's just the look of it that's not nice; it's rubbery or sticky like mucus from the nose. It's horrible.

D Any pain?

P No, not really.

D It sounds as if you've got a touch of …

Listening 2

Exercise 1

1 a It normally occurs early in the morning and sometimes late at the night or after I do any exercise, but at moment it's bad with the cold air.

   b It normally occurs early in the morning and sometimes late at night or after I do any exercise, but at the moment it's bad with the cold air.

2 a Does the breathlessness you've got have any effect on your daily activities? Your lifestyle? Your work?

   b Does breathlessness you've got have any effect on your daily activities? Your lifestyle? Your work?

3 a How many flights of stairs can you manage generally?

   b How many flights of the stairs can you manage generally?

4 a Have you had chest disease in past?

   b Have you had chest disease in the past?

5 a Is it triggered by situation or particular activity?

   b Is it triggered by a situation or particular activity?

Exercise 3

1 Yes. My father had problem with his lungs.

2 The shortness of breath came on practically immediately.

3 I can walk for quite a distance – maybe a hundred yards or so – and then I get short of breath.

4 The cold air at moment makes the breathlessness worse, so I stay at home when it's very cold.

5 I've used nebulizer.

6 I've had it for week now.

7 Does the way you lie make it worse? Or is it worse when you do the particular exercises?

Listening 3

N = Nurse, P = Patient

N There are different inhaler devices to suit different people and the one I'm going to show you how to use is this breath-activated Pressurized MDI, which stands for Metered Dose Inhaler. Are you familiar with this?

P No, not really. I've seen them, but not used one.

N Well, it's an autoinhaler, which releases a dose of the drug when a breath is taken. This means that you don't worry about breathing and hand coordination, and it means that you know that a dose has been successfully delivered.
First of all, you remove the cap and shake the inhaler several times like this.
You then prime the device by pushing this lever here right up, keeping the canister upright at the same time like this. If you find it difficult to push

the lever up by hand, you can use the edge of the table to push it against. Is this OK so far?

P Yeah. It's clear.

N OK. So you sit upright with your head up and breathe out. Then you seal your lips around the mouthpiece here. You inhale slowly and deeply. Breathe in steadily rather than quickly. When the inhaler clicks, don't stop – just continue taking a really deep breath. You won't feel the spray hitting the back of your throat although the taste in your mouth might change. Is this all OK so far?

P Yeah, fine.

N Then you remove the inhaler and hold your breath for as long as possible, mm, up to ten seconds. You then push the lever down and replace the cap. Wait a bit and then when you have recovered, take the next dose. But remember to prime it before each dose. Do you have any questions?

P No, none. It all seems very clear.

N OK, can you explain to me how to do it?

Unit 11

Listening 1

In addition to the usual differential diagnosis, in all returned travellers who present unwell, it's crucial to consider imported disease. And as tropical medicine is a specialized field, when you're unsure, seek expert advice by telephone or admit the patient.

OK, now if we turn to the next slide here, it shows what we need to ask about the history. As well as the symptoms, it's essential to find out about the area or areas travelled to, including brief stopovers, the duration of travel, immunizations received prior to travel, malaria prophylaxis, health of members of the travel party, sexual contacts whilst abroad, and medical treatment received abroad.

A full examination should be given, checking particularly for fever, jaundice, abdominal tenderness, chest signs, rashes, and lymphadenopathy.

Exact investigations depend on symptoms and examination findings, but consider FBC, thick and thin bloodfilms for malaria, LFTs, viral serology, blood culture, stool culture – ensure it is fresh – and MSU.

And on this slide we have information on malaria, which incidentally comes from a sixteenth-century Italian term – mal'aria – meaning 'foul or bad air'. There are about two thousand cases notified each year in the UK. Malaria is of course very easy to miss, one reason being that it's a great mimic, and so it can present with virtually any symptoms. It usually consists of a prodrome of headache, malaise, myalgia, and anorexia, followed by recurring fevers, rigors, and drenching sweats, which last for eight to twelve hours at a time. The examination may be normal, but one needs to look for anaemia, and jaundice with or without hepatosplenomegaly.

If we had a case of a patient, say a businessman, who had been to South America and presented with ...

Listening 2

D = Doctor, P = Patient

D You haven't had any problems for quite a while, have you?

P No, nothing serious. I've been quite lucky, really. I keep myself nice and warm, especially at this time of year, and I make sure I eat properly and drink well. I've never been a big coffee drinker, but I like a cup of tea, and I drink plenty of water as well. And even though I've had a flu jab, I keep away from people. And I always take vitamins every day without fail, so it keeps my folic acid up. My friend had leg ulcers, so I'm very careful – I'm trying to avoid that, but my hip is bad

at times, so I have to use a walking stick.

D You seem to be doing very well. You've been doing all the right things we talked about when you first became a patient here.

P Well, yes, I've done my best.

D Looking through your notes you've only had one blood transfusion, am I right?

P Yes. That was a while back. The only thing really is my hip and now this pain.

D OK, first we're going to give you painkillers.

P OK ...

Unit 12

Listening 1

A, B = Doctors

A There are many advantages to new technology. Recent medical breakthroughs like keyhole surgery are transforming the lives of patients, especially as regards the improvement in the speed of delivery of services and the speed of recovery on the part of the patient. But there's also the increased convenience for the patient in all this. Let's say we have a patient with long established diabetes, and we are able to offer a simple solution like a spray instead of injecting, then there is going to be little resistance.

B Well, the spray may not benefit every patient.

A Maybe not, but it's a step in the right direction. Can't you ever see the beneficial side of anything rather than always dwelling on the downside? Wouldn't you even feel better in yourself if you were a bit more positive?

B I'm not always negative. I'm just playing devil's advocate.

A And surely anything that makes taking medication easier is going to increase the likelihood of patients remembering to take medication and sticking to it in the long term, if needed.

B But no matter what, you have to admit that there are downsides to new technology. It's not all rosy.

A Like what, for instance?

B Well, I can think of at least two things, one being that with increased life expectancy also comes increased morbidity and not everyone wants to live with a poor quality of life. I know I wouldn't.

A You say that now, but maybe not later on, and as medical science progresses, so will quality of life for those who are living longer. I would say that by the time *we* reach *our* sixth decade, the quality of life from the medical point of view will be what it is for the average forty-year-old now.

B Maybe, and I hope you're right, but I think that there is always the danger with technology of losing sight of the patient. The information that people have is being lost as we switch on machines and the machine does the work for us. A simple example is taking blood pressure. The old sphygonometer is being replaced by digital machines and I'm not sure everyone could even read the BP correctly.

A Well, you have a point there. Deskilling is a problem, but this is all about managing change. I know it arouses debate and at times some aspects are sensitive, but I don't resist it and by and large I think the dramatic technological advances in recent years have been invaluable. And I wouldn't want to stifle change.

B Me neither. I think we agree generally but just can't agree on some of the finer detail.

A Yes, I suppose we …

Listening 2

D = Doctor, P = Patient

1 **P** Can't I just have the antibiotics I had the last time?

D Well, what you've got is different from the last time. This is a virus.

P But won't they work against viruses?

2 **P** Won't an MRI scan show if there's anything there or not?

D An MRI scan's not suitable here. It's clear from what you've said that there's nothing sinister here.

P But my friend had the same and he died of a brain tumour.

3 **P** Won't these steroids make me put on weight if I take them?

D They *can* make people add weight, but it's only a short course.

P OK.

4 **P** Isn't that new stem cell treatment available for people with strokes?

D It's still at the trial stage, I'm afraid.

P Can't my husband be part of the trial?

5 **P** Wouldn't it be better if I just stayed on this treatment for my diabetes?

D You can, but you might find this is more convenient for you. Do you want to think about it for a while?

P Yeah, OK. I'm just worried about upsetting everything, that's all.

Language spot

1 Couldn't I just keep using the same device?

2 Isn't this available on the NHS?

3 Wouldn't it be better for me just to continue with the medication?

4 Doesn't this device come with a cap on it?

5 Shouldn't my daughter be next?

6 Won't I be having the operation today either?

7 Can't I have an MRI scan?

8 Hasn't the doctor arrived yet?

9 Haven't you done that referral letter yet?

10 Didn't you say I could go home today?

11 Aren't I next on the waiting list?

Glossary

Vowels

iː	br**ee**ch	ʊ	b**oo**k	aɪ	l**i**ne
i	surger**y**	uː	m**oo**d	aʊ	g**ow**n
ɪ	d**i**sability	u	imm**u**nize	ɔɪ	av**oi**d
e	s**e**nsitive	ʌ	b**u**mp	ɪə	p**e**r**io**d
æ	par**a**medic	ɜː	c**ur**l	eə	fl**a**re
ɑː	al**ar**ming	ə	p**er**ception	ʊə	re**a**ss**ure**
ɒ	st**o**p	eɪ	**a**geing		
ɔː	w**ar**ning	əʊ	c**o**pe		

Consonants

p	h**y**pertension	f	**a**ffect	h	**h**ollow
b	**b**ronchitis	v	stop**o**ver	m	i**m**pairment
t	**t**elescope	θ	afterbi**rth**	n	ma**n**ia
d	ra**d**ical	ð	**w**ith	ŋ	alarmi**ng**
k	**c**onsent	s	di**s**locate	l	ma**l**aria
g	**g**love	z	analy**z**e	r	**r**apid **r**esponse
tʃ	dispa**tch**	ʃ	revolu**ti**on	j	**y**ourself
dʒ	bin**g**e	ʒ	conclu**s**ion	w	**w**orry

abnormal perception /æbˌnɔːml pˈsepʃn/ *n* a way of seeing or experiencing events that is not normal, especially when it is harmful or not wanted

abruptly /əˈbrʌptli/ *adv* suddenly and unexpectedly, especially in an unpleasant way

acne (vulgaris) /ˌækni vʌlˈɡɑːrɪs/ *n* a skin condition in which your face, neck, etc. is covered in pimples (= spots). Acne is common among young people.

affect /ˈæfekt/ *n* emotions or feelings, especially when considering how this influences behaviour

afterbirth /ˈɑːftəbɜːθ/ *n* the placenta and other material that comes out of a woman's body after a baby is born

ageing /ˈeɪdʒɪŋ/ *adj* becoming older

alarming /əˈlɑːmɪŋ/ *adj* causing worry and fear

analyse /ˈænəlaɪz/ *v* to study or examine something, especially by separating it into its parts, in order to understand or explain it

anosognosia /æˌnɒsɒɡˈnəʊsiə/ *n* a mental condition in which a patient is unable to recognise that they have lost a physical sense or ability

antenatal /ˌæntiˈneɪtl/ *adj* relating to the medical care given to pregnant women

anxiety /æŋˈzaɪəti/ *n* the state of feeling nervous or worried that something bad is going to happen

apathy /ˈæpəθi/ *n* the feeling of not being interested in or enthusiastic about anything

appraisal /əˈpreɪzl/ *n* a meeting in which a doctor discusses with a more senior doctor how well he or she has been doing their job; the system of holding such meetings

arrhythmia /əˈrɪðmiə/ *n* a condition in which the heart does not beat normally

atrial fibrillation /ˌeɪtriəl ˌfaɪbrɪleɪʃn/ *n* a condition in which the atria (= the two upper spaces in the heart) do not beat normally, causing the patient to develop a rapid pulse that is not regular, a common type of **arrhythmia**

avoid /əˈvɔɪd/ *v* to try not to do something because it is harmful or unpleasant

avulsion /əˈvʌlʃn/ *n* the act or process of tearing a piece from a bone by a tendon or a ligament: an avulsion fracture

baby blues /ˈbeɪbi bluːz/ *n* a depressed feeling that some women get after the birth of a baby

ball /bɔːl/ *n* (of the foot) the part underneath the big toe

bang /bæŋ/ *v* to hit a part of the body against something

barking /ˈbɑːkɪŋ/ *adj* (of a cough) very loud and produced with a lot of energy

beneficial /ˌbenɪˈfɪʃl/ *adj* improving a situation; having a helpful or useful effect

benefit from /ˈbenefit frɒm/ *v* to receive help or an advantage from something

binge /bɪndʒ/ *n* an occasion when somebody does too much of an activity they enjoy, such as eating or drinking alcohol

blemish /ˈblemɪʃ/ *n* a mark on the skin that spoils its appearance

blister /ˈblɪstə(r)/ *n* a swelling on the surface of the skin that is filled with liquid and is caused by rubbing or burning

bradykinesia /ˌbrædɪkɪˈniːziə/ *n* a condition in which a person makes unusually slow movements, often associated with Parkinson's disease

breakthrough /ˈbreɪkθruː/ *n* an important new discovery or achievement

breath-activated /ˈbreθ æktɪveɪtɪd/ *adj* (of an inhaler) releasing spray automatically when a person takes a breath

breech /briːtʃ/ *n* used to describe the position of a baby within the mother in which when it is born, the baby's feet or bottom come out first

bronchitis /brɒŋˈkaɪtɪs/ *n* an inflammation of the bronchial tubes, resulting in coughing and difficulty in breathing

bump /bʌmp/ *v* to hit something, especially a part of your body, against or on something

bystander /ˈbaɪstændə(r)/ *n* a person who sees an event, such as a crime or an accident, but who is not directly involved in it

cholesterol /kəˈlestərɒl/ *n* a substance similar to fat that is found in blood and most tissues of the body. High levels of cholesterol in the blood are associated with heart disease.

col- /kɒl-/ *prefix* relating to the colon

compelling /kəmˈpelɪŋ/ *adj* (of an idea, an argument, etc.) able to convince you that something is true

compliance /kəmˈplaɪəns/ *n* the act of following the instructions given to you by a doctor or nurse concerning your treatment, such as by taking your medicine

conclusion /kənˈkluːʒn/ *n* a judgement or a decision, made after considering all the information connected with the situation

concordance /kənˈkɔːdəns/ *n* agreement by a patient to follow a particular course of treatment after discussing the choices available to them with a doctor or nurse

consent /kənˈsent/ *n* official agreement, given by a patient to a doctor, to have a particular medical treatment such as an operation

Continuing Professional Development /kənˈtɪnjuːɪŋ prəˈfeʃnl dɪˈveləpmənt/ *n* a system for staff who are already qualified in which they receive regular training about new medical procedures connected with their job

contraindication /ˌkɒntrəˌɪndɪˈkeɪʃn/ *n* a possible reason for not giving a patient a particular drug or treatment

cope with /ˈkəʊp wɪð/ *v* to deal successfully with something difficult

crackles /ˈkræklz/ *n* small, sharp sounds that are heard when listening to the sounds within someone's body (= auscultation), often associated with emphysema (= air in the tissues)

criticism /ˈkrɪtɪsɪzəm/ *n* the act of expressing disapproval of somebody or something; a statement showing disapproval

crust /krʌst/ *n* a hard layer that covers a soft substance or liquid; a **scab**

cue /kjuː/ *n* something that you say or do in order to show somebody what you are thinking or feeling so that they may respond, give advice, etc.

curl /kɜːl/ *v* to form or make something form a curved shape, for example your toes

cysto- /ˈsɪstəʊ/ *prefix* relating to the bladder

day-case surgery /ˈdeɪ keɪs sɜːdʒəri/ *n* operations that are performed in a single day, without the need for the patient to spend the night in hospital afterwards

depend on /dɪˈpend ɒn/ *v* to rely on somebody for help or in order to do something

dermatology /ˌdɜːməˈtɒlədʒi/ *n* the area of medicine concerned with the study and treatment of skin diseases

development /dɪˈveləpmənt/ *n* **1** the process of creating something new or more advanced; a new method, product, etc.
2 a new stage in a changing situation
3 the gradual growth of something so that it becomes more advanced, stronger, etc.

disability /ˌdɪsəˈbɪləti/ *n* an inability to do something such as walk, speak, or learn normally, due to an **impairment**

disinhibition /ˌdɪsɪnhɪˈbɪʃn/ *n* the state or act of expressing your thoughts and feelings openly without concern about the opinion of other people

dislocate /ˈdɪsləkeɪt/ *v* to put a bone out of its normal position in a joint

dispatch /dɪˈspætʃ/ *v* to send a person or thing somewhere in order to do something

diuretic /ˌdaɪəˈretɪk/ *n* a substance that causes an increase in the flow of urine

DVT /ˌdiː viː ˈtiː/ *n* (deep vein thrombosis) a serious condition caused by a blood clot (= a thick mass of blood) forming in a vein

dynamic exercise /daɪˌnæmɪk ˈeksəsaɪz/ *n* physical activity in which the muscles are continuously moving, for example swimming or walking

elation /iˈleɪʃn/ *n* a feeling of great happiness and excitement

embarrassingly /ɪmˈbærəsɪŋli/ *adv* used to say that something makes you feel shy or ashamed

emotive /iˈməʊtɪv/ *adj* causing people to feel strong emotions

epidemic /ˌepɪˈdemɪk/ *n* a large number of cases of a particular disease happening at the same time in a particular community

et al /ˌet ˈæl/ *abbreviation* (used after the names of the main writers of a report, research paper, etc.) and other people not mentioned. *et al* comes from the Latin phrase *et alii/alia* = and others

evaluation /ɪˌvæljuˈeɪʃn/ *n* a judgement of the value or quality of something after thinking about it carefully

exasperated /ɪgˈzæspəreɪtɪd/ *adj* extremely annoyed, especially if you cannot do anything to improve the situation

expectation /ˌekspekˈteɪʃn/ *n* **1** a belief that something will happen because it seems likely **2** a strong belief about the way something should happen or how somebody should behave

be expecting /biː ɪkˈspektɪŋ/ *v* to be pregnant

expectoration /ɪkˌspektəˈreɪʃn/ *n* the act of coughing up material from your lungs and then spitting it out

expiratory /ˌeksˈpaɪrətri/ *adj* relating to the act of breathing out air from the lungs

faint /feɪnt/ *v* to suddenly become unconscious because not enough blood is going to your brain

fan out /ˌfæn ˈaʊt/ *v* to spread something out, like a fan

far-reaching /ˌfɑː ˈriːtʃɪŋ/ *adj* having a lot of significant effects and implications

flare up /fleər ˈʌp/ *v* (of an illness, injury, etc.) to suddenly start again or to become worse

fracture /ˈfræktʃə(r)/ *n* a break in a bone

frothy /ˈfrɒθi/ *adj* (of a liquid) full of or covered with a mass of small bubbles

frozen shoulder /frəʊzn ˈʃəʊldə(r)/ *n* a painful condition in which the shoulder joint becomes stiff and difficult to move

gait /geɪt/ *n* a way of walking

gametocyte /gəˈmiːtəsaɪt/ *n* a cell that is in the process of becoming a **gamete**

gamete /ˈgæmiːt/ *n* a male or female sex cell

get at /ˌget ˈæt/ *v* **1** to keep criticizing somebody **2** to learn or discover something

get down /ˌget ˈdaʊn/ *v* **1** to make somebody feel sad or depressed **2** to swallow or eat something, usually with difficulty

get on /ˌget ˈɒn/ *v* **1** to have a friendly relationship with somebody **2** (get on somebody's nerves) to irritate or annoy somebody

get over /ˌget ˈəʊvə(r)/ *v* **1** to return to your usual state of health after an illness **2** to deal with or gain control of a problem or difficult situation

get through to /ˌget ˈθruː tə/ *v* **1** to make contact with somebody by telephone, etc. **2** to make somebody understand or accept what you say, especially when you are trying to help them

giddy /ˈgɪdi/ *adj* feeling dizzy (= that everything is moving around and that you are going to fall)

glove /glʌv/ *v* to put on surgical gloves before an operation

gone /gɒn/ *adj* having been pregnant for the length of time mentioned

gown /gaʊn/ *v* to put on a gown (= a piece of clothing that is worn over other clothes during an operation)

groggy /ˈgrɒgi/ *adj* feeling weak and unable to think clearly because you are ill or very tired

haemolyze /ˈhiːməlaɪz/ *v* to destroy red blood cells by causing them to break open and release their haemoglobin; to be destroyed in this way

hairline /ˈheəlaɪn/ *n* a very thin crack or line in the surface of a bone: a hairline fracture

handicap /ˈhændikæp/ *n* in inability to do certain things such as do a particular job, get an education, etc., because of a **disability**

hazardous /ˈhæzədəs/ *adj* dangerous, especially to somebody's health or safety

heel /hiːl/ *n* the raised part of the inside of the hand where it joins the wrist

hernia /ˈhɜːniə/ *n* a condition in which part of an organ is pushed through the body wall around it

herniorrhaphy /ˌhɜːniˈɒrəfi/ *n* an operation to repair a **hernia**

high /haɪ/ *n* the highest level or largest number of something

hoarse /hɔːrs/ *adj* (of a cough, a voice, etc.) sounding rough and unpleasant, because of a sore throat

hobble /ˈhɒbl/ *v* to walk with difficulty, especially because your feet or legs hurt

hollow /ˈhɒləʊ/ *adj* (of a cough) making a low, empty sound

host /həʊst/ *n* an animal or a plant on which another living thing (= a parasite) lives and feeds

hypertension /ˌhaɪpəˈtenʃn/ *n* blood pressure that is higher than is normal

hystero- /ˈhɪstərəʊ/ *prefix* relating to the uterus

impacted /ɪmˈpæktɪd/ *adj* used to describe a type of fracture in which the two broken ends of the bone are pushed into each other

impairment /ɪmˈpeəmənt/ *n* a condition in which you are not able to use a part of your body or brain normally

impromptu /ɪmˈprɒmptjuː/ *adj, adv* done without preparation or planning

inconsolable /ˌɪnkənˈsəʊləbl/ *adj* extremely sad and unable to accept help or comfort

ingenious /ɪnˈdʒiːniəs/ *adj* (of a device, a plan, a method, etc.) very suitable for a particular purpose and using clever new ideas

inspiratory /ˌɪnsˈpaɪrətri/ *adj* relating to the act of breathing in air to the lungs

intussusception /ˌɪntəsəˈsepʃn/ *n* a painful condition, most common among young children, in which a section of the intestine becomes folded within itself with the result that it becomes blocked

itch /ɪtʃ/ *v* to have an uncomfortable feeling on your skin that makes you want to scratch it; to make your skin feel like this

job specification /dʒɒb ˌspesɪfɪˈkeɪʃn/ *n* a description of the skills, knowledge, and experience that are required to do a particular job

keep /ˌkiːp/ *v* to continue doing something

land /lænd/ *v* to come down to the ground after falling, jumping, or being thrown

laparo- /ˈlæpərəʊ/ *prefix* relating to the abdomen

laparotomy /ˌlæpəˈrɒtəmi/ *n* a procedure in which a cut is made in the abdomen, usually in order to examine the organs inside

lie /laɪ/ *n* the position in which a baby is lying within the mother

life cycle /'laɪf saɪkl/ *n* the series of changes in the life of an animal, plant, etc.

lifestyle /'laɪfstaɪl/ *n* the way in which a person lives, including their work, hobbies, diet, physical activity, etc.

line /laɪn/ *n* a course of treatment

longitudinal /ˌlɒŋɡɪ'tjuːdɪnl/ *adj* (of a baby within the mother) lying in an upward or downward position rather than across the mother's body

malaise /mə'leɪz/ *n* a general feeling of being ill

malaria /mə'leəriə/ *n* a disease that causes fever, caused by a blood parasite that is passed to people by the bite of a mosquito

mania /'meɪniə/ *n* a mental illness in which a person behaves in a very excited and active way and may also have exaggerated beliefs about their abilities

marche à petit pas /ˌmɑːʃ ə pəti 'pɑː/ *n* a way of walking in which the person takes unusually small steps, often associated with Parkinson's disease

masto- / mammo- /'mæstəʊ/ /'mæməʊ/ *prefix* relating to the breast

MDI /ˌem diː 'aɪ/ *n* (metered dose inhaler) a type of inhaler that releases a specific amount of medicine each time it is used

mean /miːn/ *v* **1** to intend to do something **2** to involve; to have as a consequence

membrane /'membreɪn/ *n* a thin layer of skin or tissue that connects or covers organs or other parts inside the body

mental state examination /ˌmentl 'steɪt ɪɡzæmɪˌneɪʃn/ *n* an interview between a doctor and a patient in order to judge the patient's present mental condition

merozoite /ˌmerə'zəʊaɪt/ *n* a stage in the **life cycle** of the parasite that causes **malaria**. Merozoites are formed in large numbers by a **schizont** and either become another schizont or a sex cell (= **gamete**).

milestone /'maɪlstəʊn/ *n* a very important stage or event in the development of something

mitral stenosis /ˌmaɪtrəl stɪ'nəʊsɪs/ *n* a condition in which the mitral valve

(= the opening that connects the left atrium and the left ventricle of the heart) becomes more narrow than is normal

mood /muːd/ *n* the way you are feeling at a particular time

morbidity /mɔː'bɪdəti/ *n* the number of people who have a particular illness

morning sickness /'mɔːnɪŋ sɪknəs/ *n* the need to vomit that some women feel when they are pregnant, often only in the morning

mortality /mɔː'tæləti/ *n* the number of people who die from a particular illness

negotiate /nɪ'ɡəʊʃieɪt/ *v* to agree something by formal discussion

nephro- /'nefrəʊ/ *prefix* relating to the kidney(s)

notifiable /'nəʊtɪfaɪəbl/ *adj* (of a disease) so serious that it must be reported to the authorities

objectionable /əb'dʒekʃənəbl/ *adj* unpleasant or offensive

offensive /ə'fensɪv/ *adj* extremely unpleasant

on edge /ɒn 'edʒ/ *adj* to be nervous, excited, or bad-tempered

on top of the world /ɒn ˌtɒp əv ðə 'wɜːld/ *adj* very happy or proud

pandemic /pæn'demɪk/ *n* a serious disease that spreads over a whole region or a large part of the world

paramedic /ˌpærə'medɪk/ *n* a person whose job involves giving emergency medical treatment to sick or injured people in their home, at the scene of an accident, etc., before they are taken to hospital

patch /pætʃ/ *n* a small area of something that is different from the area around it

perforated appendix /pɜːfəreɪtɪd ə'pendɪks/ *n* a serious condition in which the appendix bursts after becoming infected and then swollen

pericarditis /ˌperɪkɑː'daɪtɪs/ *n* a serious inflammation of the pericardium (= the thin layer of tissue surrounding the heart)

period /'pɪəriəd/ *n* the flow of blood each month from the body of a woman who is not pregnant

persuasion /pə'sweɪʒn/ *n* the act of convincing somebody to do something

persuasive /pə'sweɪsɪv/ *adj* able to persuade somebody to do or believe something

pick at /'pɪk ət/ *v* to touch something several times with your nails or fingers, especially by repeatedly removing small pieces of it

pick up /ˌpɪk 'ʌp/ *v* **1** to take hold of something and lift it up **2** to start again; continue

play with /'pleɪ wɪð/ *v* to keep touching or moving something

POP /ˌpiː əʊ 'piː/ *n* (plaster of paris) a white powder that becomes hard when it is mixed with water and left to dry. POP is used to make plaster casts (= a solid case that is put on a person's body in order to cover and protect a broken bone); a cast made of this material

pre-eclampsia /priː ɪ'klæmpsiə/ *n* a condition in which a pregnant woman has high blood pressure, which can become serious if it is not treated

productive /prə'dʌktɪv/ *adj* (of a cough) producing **sputum** or mucus (= a thick liquid that is produced in parts of the body, such as the nose)

prone to sth /'prəʊn tə/ *adj* likely to suffer from something, such as a particular illness

psychosocial /ˌsaɪkəʊ'səʊʃl/ *adj* concerning the mental and social aspects of something and how they influence each other

purpura /pɜː'pjʊərə/ *n* an area of red or purple spots on the skin, caused by bleeding underneath the surface of the skin

purulent /'pjʊərələnt/ *adj* containing or producing pus (= a thick yellowish liquid that is produced in an infected wound)

radical /'rædɪkl/ *adj* new and very different from what is usually done

rapid response /ˌræpɪd rɪ'spɒns/ *n* the act or process of dealing with a medical emergency quickly

rapport /ræ'pɔː(r)/ *n* a friendly relationship in which people understand each other very well

reckless /'rekləs/ *adj* showing a lack of care about the danger or the consequences of your actions

reduction /rɪ'dʌkʃn/ *n* the act or process of returning a part of the body to its normal position, for example after a **hernia**, by performing an operation or other medical procedure

rehabilitation /ˌriːəˌbɪlɪ'teɪʃn/ *n* the process in which a person learns to have a normal life again after they have been very ill or had a serious injury

resect /rɪ'sekt/ *v* to cut out part of an organ or a piece of tissue from the body

revolution /ˌrevə'luːʃn/ *n* a major change in methods, ideas, etc. that affects many people

rigidity /rɪ'dʒɪdəti/ *n* the state of being stiff and difficult to move or bend

rigor /'rɪgə(r)/ *n* a sudden attack of shivering (= shaking of the body), accompanied by a feeling of coldness and a rapid rise in body temperature, usually indicating the start of a fever

rupture /'rʌptʃə(r)/ *v* to burst or break apart something inside the body; to be broken or to burst apart

safety net /'seɪfti net/ *n* used to describe any arrangement that is intended to protect a patient and prevent problems from developing after they finish consulting a doctor or having treatment

scab /skæb/ *n* a hard layer of dried blood that forms over a cut as it heals

scab over /'skæb əʊvə(r)/ *v* to form a **scab**

schizont /'skaɪzɒnt/ *also* /'ʃaɪzɒnt/ *n* a stage in the **life cycle** of the parasite that causes **malaria**, during which it reproduces itself many times by dividing to form new cells (= **merozoites**)

scrub up /ˌskrʌb 'ʌp/ *v* (of a doctor, nurse, etc.) to wash your hands and arms before performing an operation

seizure /'siːʒə(r)/ *n* a sudden attack of an illness, such as epilepsy, in which a person becomes unconscious and their body shakes violently; = a fit

sensitive /'sensətɪv/ *adj* **1** (of a subject) needing to be treated carefully because it may offend or upset people **2** (of people) easily offended or upset

shuffling /'ʃʌflɪŋ/ *adj* (of the way somebody walks) slowly without lifting your feet completely off the ground; SEE **marche à petit pas**

sickle-cell anaemia /ˌsɪkl sel ə'niːmiə/ *n* a serious form of anaemia, mostly affecting people of African origin, in which the red blood cells lose their normal shape when oxygen levels are low

simple /'sɪmpl/ *adj* (of a fracture) involving a break of the bone but with little damage to the surrounding skin and muscle

slip (over) /'slɪp ˌəʊvə(r)/ *v* to slide a short distance by accident so that you fall or nearly fall

small of the back /ˌsmɔːl əv ðə 'bæk/ *n* the lower part of the back where it curves in

small talk /'smɔːl tɔːk/ *n* polite conversation about ordinary or unimportant subjects, for example in order to make a patient feel relaxed

smash /smæʃ/ *v* to break something violently into many pieces; to be broken in this way

SOCRATES /'sɒkrətiːz/ *n* used as a way of remembering how to judge the nature of a patient's pain. Each letter of SOCRATES refers to a word which relates to a question, the words are: **S**ite, **O**nset, **C**haracter, **R**adiation, **A**ssociations, **T**iming of pain/duration, **E**xacerbating/Relieving factors, **S**everity

soil /sɔɪl/ *v* to accidentally release solid waste from your body onto your clothes, bed sheets, etc.

spiral /'spaɪrəl/ *adj* (of a fracture) caused by twisting the bone so that it breaks

spontaneously /spɒn'teɪniəsli/ *adv* happening naturally, without the need for medical treatment or assistance

sporozoite /ˌspɒrə'zəʊaɪt/ *n* a stage in the **life cycle** of the parasite that causes **malaria**. Sporozoites form within the body of a mosquito which then passes them to humans where they travel to the liver cells to form a **schizont**.

sputum /'spjuːtəm/ *n* thick liquid from the throat or lungs that is coughed up because of disease, etc. In non-medical situations, sputum is often called phlegm /flem/.

squash /skwɒʃ/ *v* to press or crush something so that it becomes damaged or changes shape

statin /'stætɪn/ *n* a type of drug that helps to lower **cholesterol**

stop /stɒp/ *v* to prevent somebody from doing something

stopover /'stɒpəʊvə(r)/ *n* a short stay somewhere between two parts of a journey

straighten /'streɪtn/ *v* to become straight; to make something straight

stub /stʌb/ *v* to hurt your toe by accidentally hitting it against something hard

stumble /'stʌmbl/ *v* to fall or almost fall while you are walking or running

sweetened /'swiːtnd/ *adj* (of food or a drink) made to taste sweeter by adding sugar, etc.

telescope /'telɪskəʊp/ *v* (of the different parts of something) to slide within each other

tenacious /tə'neɪʃəs/ *adj* sticky and difficult to pull apart

the Pill /ðə 'pɪl/ *n* the contraceptive pill (= a pill that some women take to prevent them becoming pregnant)

thread /θred/ *n* an idea that connects the different parts of a conversation, argument, etc.

thrombolysis /ˌθrɒm'bɒlɪsɪs/ *n* the act or process of dissolving a blood clot (= a thick mass of blood)

tickly /'tɪkli/ *adj* (of a cough) producing an irritating sensation on your throat that makes you want to cough

tingling /'tɪŋglɪŋ/ *n* an uncomfortable feeling in a part of your body as if a lot of small sharp points are pushing into it

tolerate /'tɒləreɪt/ *v* to be able to be affected by a drug without being harmed

travellers' diarrhoea /ˌtrævələz daɪəˈrɪə/ *n* an illness in which you pass solid waste from your body frequently, and in liquid form, and which is developed while travelling in a foreign country

tremor /ˈtremə(r)/ *n* a slight shaking movement in a part of your body, often associated with Parkinson's disease

trend /trend/ *n* a general direction in which a situation is changing or developing

trip (over/up) | trip (over/on sth) /ˈtrɪp ˌəʊvə(r)/ /-ˌʌp/ /-ˌɒn/ *v* to catch your foot on something and fall or almost fall

try (for a baby) /traɪ/ *v* to attempt to conceive

twist /twɪst/ *v* to injure part of your body, especially your ankle, wrist, or knee, by bending it in an awkward way

twitch /twɪtʃ/ *v* (of a person's body) to make a sudden quick movement, especially one that you cannot control

uncooperative /ˌʌnkəʊˈɒpərətɪv/ *adj* not willing to be helpful to other people or do what they ask

uneasy /ʌnˈiːzi/ *adj* feeling worried or unhappy about a particular situation

unequivocal /ˌʌnɪˈkwɪvəkl/ *adj* expressing your opinion or intention very clearly and firmly

unhygienic /ˌʌnhaɪˈdʒiːnɪk/ *adj* not clean and therefore likely to cause disease or infection

unjustifiable /ʌnˈdʒʌstɪfaɪəbl/ *adj* (of an action) impossible to excuse or accept because there is no good reason for it

unpeeled /ʌnˈpiːld/ *adj* (of a fruit or vegetable) with a skin that has not been removed

variolation /ˌveəriəˈlaɪʃn/ *n* (historical) the practice of deliberately giving somebody a small amount of the smallpox (= variola) virus so that they cannot catch this disease in future

vesicle /ˈvesɪkl/ *n* a small **blister** filled with clear liquid, associated with skin conditions such as eczema

warning /ˈwɔːnɪŋ/ *n* an instruction telling somebody what to do or what not to do

warning sign /ˈwɔːnɪŋ saɪn/ *n* a change in a person's health or behaviour that indicates that they may have a particular illness; = a prodrome

wet /wet/ **1** *v* to urinate by accident **2** *adj* (of weather) rain

wheal *also* **weal** /wiːl/ *n* a sore red swelling on the skin, associated with skin conditions such as urticaria

woozy /ˈwuːzi/ *adj* feeling unsteady and confused

worry about /ˈwʌri əbaʊt/ *v* to keep thinking about unpleasant things that might happen or about problems that you have

wryneck /ˈraɪnek/ *n* a condition affecting the neck muscles which causes the neck to turn so that eventually the head is permanently held to one side; = torticollis

OXFORD
UNIVERSITY PRESS

Great Clarendon Street, Oxford OX2 6DP

Oxford University Press is a department of the University of Oxford.
It furthers the University's objective of excellence in research, scholarship,
and education by publishing worldwide in

Oxford New York

Auckland Cape Town Dar es Salaam Hong Kong Karachi
Kuala Lumpur Madrid Melbourne Mexico City Nairobi
New Delhi Shanghai Taipei Toronto

With offices in

Argentina Austria Brazil Chile Czech Republic France Greece
Guatemala Hungary Italy Japan Poland Portugal Singapore
South Korea Switzerland Thailand Turkey Ukraine Vietnam

OXFORD and OXFORD ENGLISH are registered trade marks of
Oxford University Press in the UK and in certain other countries

© Oxford University Press 2010

ISBN: 978 0 19 456956 9

Printed in China

ACKNOWLEDGEMENTS

Illustrations by: Julian Baker pp.19, 31, 45, 49, 62, 70, 79, 91, 96, 101, 102 (map); www.cartoonstock.com
p.87; Mark Duffin pp.16 (pan fire, knife, tin can, plug), 35; Melvyn Evans pp.42, 71; Joy Gosney pp.38,
112 (Pandora's box); Andy Hammond p.104 (cartoon); Ian Moores pp.21, 56, 104 (patient care); Oxford
Handbook of Psychiatry p.43 (graph); Oxford Handbook of Geriatric Medicine p.50; Oxford Handbook
of Clinical Medicine 7 p.57 (lesions), 82 (ECGs), 6th edition p.95 (peak flow chart); Oxford Handbook
of Renal Medicine p.96 (diagram); Tony Sigley pp.5, 12, 25, 2, 30, 37, 39, 77, 84, 109.

Cover image courtesy of: Masterfile

The Publisher would like to thank the following for their kind permission to reproduce photographs: age
fotostock p.14 (X-ray of fractured toe/Dinodia); Alamy Images pp.13 (Leg in plaster/Helene Rogers),
Alamy Images p.14 (Abraham Colles); Alamy Images p.16 (Coloured x-ray); 18 (Arm in plaster/Rodger
Tamblyn), 20 (Runner with pulled muscle/Dennis MacDonald), 20 (Painful hamstring/John Fryer),
22 (Blistered hand/JHP Adults), 23 (man with bad back/vario images GmbH & Co.KG), 28 (antenatal
class/Bubbles Photolibrary), 29 (antenatal ultrasonic scan/peter haslund karlsson), Alamy Images
p.41 (Post-natal depression/AJ Photo); Alamy Images p.44 (Aerobics exercise class/John Cole); 47
(Rehabilitation ward/Ilene MacDonald), 57 (Senior citizens fitness class/INSADCO Photography),
61 (Close-up of hands/Horizon International Images Limited), Alamy Images p.66 (Lichen planus/
James Stevenson); Alamy Images p.68 (Itchy skin/Lea Paterson); 69 (acne rosacea/Hercules
Robinson), 72 (Nurse/Geomphotography), Alamy Images p.75 (Hernia operation/Mark Thomas;
Alamy Images p.80 (Medical training/Sam Ogden); 90 (Flying pollen/blickwinkel), 90 (Dusty building
site/FogStock), Alamy Images p.96 (Inhaler/Gustoimages); Alamy Images p.106 (Nanorobot/Roger
Harris); 114 (Psoriasis/Hercules Robinson); Corbis pp.4 (Air ambulance medics/David Spurdens), 9
(Mobile Emergency Defibrillator/Paul Seheult/Eye Ubiquitous), 36 (Ernest Hemingway/Bettmann),
36 (Samuel Beckett/Hulton-Deutsch Collection), 36 (Audrey Hepburn/John Springer Collection), 36
(Marilyn Monroe/Bettmann), 44 (Researchers wearing old age simulation devices/TWPhoto), Corbis
p.46 (Elderly woman walking/Joan Comalat/age fotostock); 48 (Swimming exercise class/Ronnie
Kaufman), 53 (Deconstruction work/Kathrin Brunnhofer/epa), 58 (Newly opened Roman box/
Reuters), 59 (Endoscopic surgery training/John Madere), 66 (Woman with freckles/Patrik Giardino),
66 (Eczema/Lester V. Bergman), 69 (Discarded medication/Ursula Klawitter), 72 (Medicine cabinet/
George B. Diebold), Corbis p.74 (Surgeon preparing for surgery/Art Becker/Art Becker Photography/
Flirt Collection); 98 (Women planting rice/Frans Lanting), 112 (Frankenstein's Monster/Bettmann);
Getty Images pp.20 (Injured rugby player Shane McDonald), 40 (Sigmund Freud), 66 (Sunburn/Peter
Cade), 106 (Pacemakers); OUP pp.32 (woman/Photodisc), 34 (Birthday celebrations/image100), 46
(James Parkinson/CJ Sword), 54 (Skier/Photodisc), 86 (scales/Digital Vision), 86 (cyclists/Photodisc),
86 (salad/Image Source), 86 (ashtray/BananaStock), 98 (Crowd/Photodisc), 98 (Aircraft landing/
Digital Vision), 100 (tomatoes/Photodisc), 100 (strawberries/Photodisc), 100 (grapes/Ingram), 100 (ice
cream/Mark Mason), 107 (Couple talking at table/Photodisc), 110 (Medicine/Photodisc); Photolibrary
pp.4 (Paramedics/White), 6 (Using a mobile phone/Glow Images), 6 (Doctor with patient/Index Stock
Imagery), 7 (X-ray/Scott Camazine/Phototake Science), 8 (Cyclist/Nicole Hill/Rubberball), 15 (Doctor
smiling/Seth Joel/White), 20 (Dehydrated/BlueMoon Images/Bluemoon Stock Inc.), 24 (School sports
day/GoGo Images), 28 (Woman in doctor's office/Monkey Business Images Ltd/Stockbroker), 33
(Doctor with patient/Asia Images Group), 34 (Cutting umbilical cord/Herve Gyssels/Photononstop),
44 (Elderly woman in chair/Image Source), 66 (Psoriasis/Medicimage), 67 (Allergy test/Image Source),
74 (Day surgery unit/Image Source), 81 (Group of doctors studying/Javier Larrea/age fotostock), 82
(Mid section view of young man/ImageDJ), 86 (Pouring salt/Banana Stock), 87 (Measuring blood
pressure/Claude Cortier/AGE Photostock), 88 (Doctor with patient/Hervé Gyssels/Photononstop), 88
(Woman taking pills/Stockbroker), 90 (Living room/David George/Red Cover), 90 (Woman sneezing/
Martin Leigh/OSF), 90 (Crowded public transport/White), 90 (Waiting room/Science Photo Library
RF), 93 (Testing for TB/CDC/Phototake Science), 98 (Spa room/MAISANT Ludovic/Hemis), 98 (Blue
Poison Dart Frog/Chris Mattison/age fotostock), 99 (Mosquito biting/P&R Fotos/age fotostock), 100
(Medical seminar/Banana Stock), 100 (Star fruit/Burke Triolo/Brand X Pictures), 100 (Kebab/Ciaran
Griffin/White), 100 (Cola/FoodCollection), 103 (Blood transfusion/Yoav Levy/Phototake Science),
106 (Blood Pressure Sphygmomanometer/Ron Chapple Stock/Photolibrary RF), 110 (MRI Scanner/
Corbis), 110 (Ultrasound Machine/Corbis), 110 (Lumbar Puncture/LAURENT/B HOP AME/BSIP Medical),
112 (Stem cell illustration/GILLES/BSIP Medical); PunchStock p.7 (Battery/Photodisc); Rex Features
pp.4 (London Motorcycle Paramedic/ITV), 4 (Paramedic using a bicycle), 106 (Futuristic ambulance);
Science Photo Library pp.16 (Lateral X-Ray of the Elbow/Living Art Enterprises, LLC), 16 (Fractured
fibula x-ray/Athenais, ISM), 16 (Fractured pelvis, x-ray/Du Cane Medical Imaging Ltd), 28 (Obstetric
consultation/Ian Hooton), 28 (Newborn baby/Keith/Custom Medical Stock Photo), 40 (Emil Kraepelin/
National Library of Medicine), 66 (Vitiligo skin disorder/Maria Platt-Evans), 66 (Rash/Dr p. Marazzi),
66 (Scabies/Dr p. Marazzi), 69 (Impetigo/Dr p. Marazzi), 71 (Acne vulgaris/St. Bartholomew's Hospital),
71 (Acne vulgaris/Dr p. Marazzi), 71 (Acne on chin/Dr p. Marazzi), 74 (Hospital recovery room/Simon
Fraser), 76 (X-ray of appendix and colon/Lunagrafix), 78 (Dermoid ovarian cyst/ISM), 80 (Removal of
an ovarian cyst/Dr Najeeb Layyous), 82 (X-ray of enlarged heart/Dr p. Marazzi), 92 (X-ray of pulmonary
embolism/Zephyr), 93 (TB Skin Test/Martin M. Rotker), 93 (Tuberculosis diagnosis/Andy Crump, TDR,
WHO), 93 (Testing for lung diseases/Arno Massee), 95 (Lung function test/Coneyl Jay), 102 (Sickle cell
anaemia SEM), 106 (Artificial hand/Volker Steger), 106 (Cell division/Dr Paul Andrews, University of
Dundee), 108 (Bone bioceramic/Klaus Guldbrandsen), 110 (Heart surgery/Volkar Steger), 110 (X-ray
machines/Gustoimages), 110 (Medical prescription/Cristina Pedrazzini), 110 (Acupuncture/Tek Image),
111 (Stem cell), 113 (Albert Szent-Gyorgi), 114 (atopic eczema), 115 (Swollen leg/Dr p. Marazzi), 115
(venous leg ulcer/Dr p. Marazzi); University of Wisconsin-Madison Archives p.40 (Courtesy University
of Wisconsin-Madison Archives); Wellcome Trust Medical Photographic Library pp.34 (Hospital birth
room), 74 (Sutures on a manikin).

*The author and publisher are grateful to those who have given permission to reproduce the following extracts
and adaptations of copyright material:* pp.8 and 9 Extracts from 'Square Mile cycle-paramedics become
the new City-slickers', 14 August 2006, from www.londonambulance.nhs.uk. Reproduced by
permission; p.10 Extract from 'Guidelines on Continuing Professional Development' by Jacky
Hanson and Henry Guly, from www.collemergencymed.ac.uk. Reproduced by permission; pp.16,
17, 18 Extracts from 'Accidents and their Prevention' by Dr M Preston, from www.patient.co.uk.
Reproduced by permission; p.24 Extract from Coalter, F (2009) 'Physical fitness and health', Value
of Sport Monitor, Sport England/UK Sport. Reproduced by permission; p.32 Extract from 'Antenatal
Classes' from www.nct.org.uk. Reproduced by permission; p.34 Extract from 'Third Stage of Labour'
from www.nct.org.uk. Reproduced by permission; p.40 From Oxford Handbook of Psychiatry by
Semple, D, Oxford University Press 2006. Reproduced by permission; p.47 From Oxford Handbook
of Geriatric Medicine by Bowler, L et al., Oxford University Press 2006. Reproduced by permission;
p.52 From Oxford Handbook of Emergency Medicine 3rd Edition by Wyatt, J. p. et al., Oxford
University Press 2006. Reproduced by permission; p.54 Extract from 'The Big Question: Is skiing
now so dangerous that speed limits should be imposed?' by Jamie Buckley, 15 January 2009, The
Independent. Reproduced by permission; p.55 From 'Involving fathers in maternity care: best
practice' by Jeremy Davies © The Royal College of Midwives 2009. All Rights Reserved. Reproduced
by permission; p.56 From 'Brain pattern associated with genetic risk of Obsessive Compulsive
Disorder' by Genevieve Maul, 26 November 2007, from www.admin.cam.ac.uk. Reproduced by
permission; p.57 From 'More seniors-only fitness centres popping up', 19 June 2007. Reproduced
by permission of The Press Association; p.58 From 'Roman face cream found at London temple
site' by Paul Peachey, 29 July 2003, The Independent. Reproduced by permission; p.59 From 'New
training method helps surgeons evaluate their own minimally invasive surgery skills', 12 January
2009, Delft University of Technology www.tudelft.nl. Reproduced by permission; p.60 From 'Heart's
Surplus Energy May Help Power Pacemakers, Defibrillators'. Reprinted with permission, http://
americanheart.mediaroom.com/index.php?s=43&item=547 © 2009, American Heart Association,
Inc.; p.61 From Oxford Handbook of Respiratory Medicine by Chapman, S et al. Oxford University
Press 2006. Reproduced by permission; p.62 From Oxford Handbook of Expedition and Wilderness
Medicine by Johnson, C. Oxford University Press 2008. Reproduced by permission; p.63 From 'Smart
fabrics make clever (medical) clothing' from ICT Results, http://cordis.europa.eu/ictresults; p.70
From Oxford Handbook of Clinical Examination and Practical Skills by Thomas, J et al. Oxford
University Press 2008. Reproduced by permission; p.78 From 'Ovarian Cyst' from www.patient.
co.uk. Reproduced by permission; p.79 From Oxford Handbook of Clinical Medicine 7th Edition
by Longmore, M. Oxford University Press 2007. Reproduced by permission; p.86 From 'High Blood
Pressure – Hypertension' by Dr Richard Maddison, 2008, from www.bcpa.co.uk , The British Cardiac
Patients Association. Reproduced by permission; pp.90, 91 From Oxford Handbook of Clinical
Examination and Practical Skills by Thomas, J et al., Oxford University Press 2008. Reproduced
by permission; p.99 From Oxford Handbook of General Practice 2nd Edition by Pencheon, D et
al., Oxford University Press 2006. Reproduced by permission; pp.100, 101, 102, 103 From Oxford
Handbook of Tropical Medicine 3rd Edition by Eddleston, M et al., Oxford University Press 2008.
Reproduced by permission; p.111 From 'Stem Cell Transplant' from www.patient.co.uk. Reproduced
by permission; p.111 From 'Sue Gyford: A new vision of hope for the blind' by Sue Gyford, 21 January
2009, from http://news.scotsman.com. Reproduced by permission; p.111 From 'Stem Cell Basics' by
National Institutes of Health, from http://stemcells.nih.gov.

Sources: pp.5, 6, 12, 15 Oxford Handbook of Emergency Medicine 3rd Edition by Wyatt, J. p. et al.,
Oxford University Press 2006; pp.22, 45, 47, 85, 90, 93 Oxford Handbook of Clinical Medicine 7th
Edition by Longmore, M et al., Oxford University Press 2007; pp.28, 29 Oxford Handbook of Clinical
Specialities 7th Edition by Collier, Longmore and Brinsden, Oxford University Press 2006; pp.39, 41,
42 Oxford Handbook of Psychiatry by Semple, D, Oxford University Press 2006; p.50 2004 figures
from Eurostat; p.66 Oxford Handbook of Clinical Examination and Practical Skills by Thomas,
J et al., Oxford University Press 2008; p.78 Oxford Handbook of Clinical Surgery 3rd Edition by
McLatchie, G et al., Oxford University Press 2007; pp.82, Oxford Handbook of General Practice 2nd
Edition by Pencheon, D et al., Oxford University Press 2006; pp.91, 92, 93, 94 Oxford Handbook
of Respiratory Medicine by Chapman, S, Oxford University Press 2006; p.98 Oxford Handbook of
Public Health Practice 2nd Edition by Pencheon, D, et al., Oxford University Press; p.104 Oxford
Handbook of Tropical Medicine 3rd Edition by Eddlestone, M et al., Oxford University Press 2008

*Although every effort has been made to trace and contact copyright holders before publication, this has not been
possible in some cases. We apologize for any apparent infringement of copyright and if notified, the publisher will
be pleased to rectify any errors or omissions at the earliest opportunity.*

The author and publisher would like to thank the following people who assisted in the development of this title:
Dr Mark Fenton MA (Oxon) PhD MB BS MRCP(UK), Consultant Cardiologist, Kent and Canterbury
Hospital, East Kent Hospitals Trust; Dean Wang, Escola d'Idiomes, University of Vic, Spain.

Special thanks are also due to: Eileen Flannigan (author: Grammar Reference), Ben Francis (author:
Glossary, Website), Anna Gunn, Diane Winkleby, and Lewis Lansford for his considerable editorial
support and guidance.